$6.95

W9-AAK-801

OTHER VOLUMES IN
EXERCISES IN DIAGNOSTIC RADIOLOGY

Published

and

ADVANCED EXERCISES IN DIAGNOSTIC RADIOLOGY

Published

Forthcoming

Advanced
EXERCISES IN DIAGNOSTIC RADIOLOGY

10

THE URINARY TRACT

ANTHONY WALSH, F.R.C.S.I.
Department of Urology
Jervis Street Hospital
Dublin, Ireland

JAMES G. McNULTY, F.R.C.R.
Department of Radiology
Jervis Street Hospital
Dublin, Ireland

W. B. SAUNDERS COMPANY • PHILADELPHIA • LONDON • TORONTO   1977

W. B. Saunders   West Washington Square
Philadelphia, PA   19105

1 St. Anne's Road
Eastbourne, East Sussex BN21 3UN, England

1 Goldthorne Avenue
Toronto, Ontario M8Z 5T9, Canada

THE URINARY TRACT
Advanced Exercises in Diagnostic Radiology—Volume 10   ISBN   0-7216-9112-9

Last digit is the print number: 9   8   7   6   5   4   3   2   1

PREFACE

This volume is part of a continuing series. The most idle glance will inform the reader that the overall text owes a great deal to the inspiration and example of Lucy Frank Squire; it is dedicated to her in recognition of her genius as a teacher.

In this volume we have attempted to provide the basic radiological approach to urological problems — to show how radiology must be integrated with the overall clinical approach to the patient and his disorder.

In many modern institutions the problems described in this book would have been studied by ultrasound and scanning techniques. These relatively new techniques have been deliberately omitted from this text. Diagnostic ultrasound has already been the subject of a separate volume in this series.

We have not attempted to present a complete acount of the radiology of the urinary tract; our hope has been to illustrate the ways in which radiology can illuminate diagnosis in urology.

All of the patients depicted in *The Urinary Tract* are real, although, obviously, their names have been changed.

We would like to thank our colleagues Dr. J. Toland and Mr. Peter McLean for contributing cases to this book. We would also like to record our deep appreciation of the technical skill and human forbearance of the Publishers, the W. B. Saunders Company, to whom this work owes so much.

ANTHONY WALSH
JAMES G. McNULTY

CONTENTS

Penny Stone, now age 11, is brought by her mother to the emergency room because she has swallowed a large English coin. As it is a big coin, you can expect to find it lodged in *Penny's* esophagus but a chest film is normal. You request a plain film of the abdomen (Fig. 1). What are your observations?

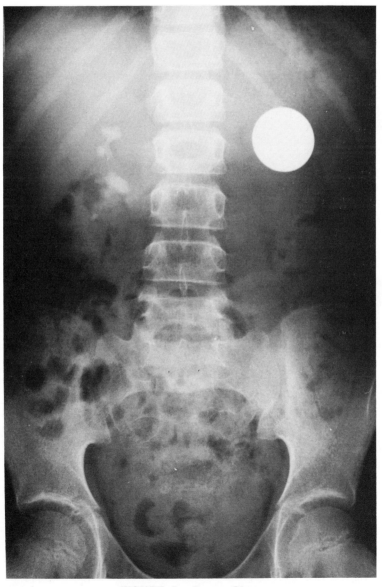

FIGURE 1. Penny Stone

The coin is in **Penny's** stomach. But to your great surprise there is also a staghorn calculus in the right kidney. *Penny* had her appendix removed six years previously but has never had any other illness.

It is not uncommon to find large stones like this in an x-ray done for some unrelated reason, especially in barium studies requested as part of the work-up of a patient with an ill-defined dyspepsia.

What are you going to do about *Penny* now?

Penny Stone's urinalysis revealed a trace of albumin and a few white cells but culture was sterile. The intravenous pyelogram that you requested (Fig. 2) shows good function on both sides but there is considerable dilatation of the calyces of the right kidney, owing to obstruction caused by the calculus.

Incidentally, you notice that the coin has gone: Like the majority of foreign bodies that enter the stomach, it was passed naturally.

Penny's calculi were removed by pyelolithotomy. You request serum calcium and uric acid levels and also tests to exclude renal tubular acidosis. You also have the urine tested for cystine: Cystine stones are not common, but it is very important to identify them because they can be prevented and because they are familial.

All these tests are negative. We do not know the cause of *Penny's* stone but at least she was fortunate that for once she put a coin in her mouth instead of in her purse. If the calculus had not been discovered, the right kidney might have been destroyed before any symptoms developed.

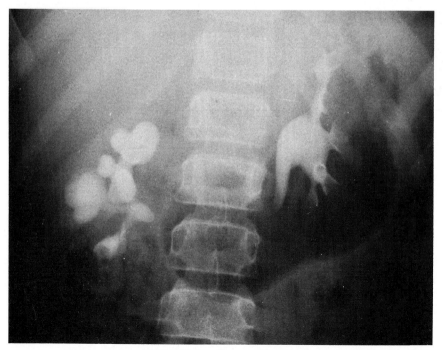

FIGURE 2. Penny Stone

John Dory is a 64 year old retired stockbroker who is referred by his family doctor for investigation because of recent severe pain in the left loin. *Mr. Dory* tells you that his right kidney was removed for carcinoma 20 years previously, and that he had a severe myocardial infarction 8 years ago.

Physical examination reveals considerable arteriosclerosis and a blood pressure of 180/100, but nothing else remarkable. Urinalysis is negative except for a trace of albumin and a very few red and white blood cells. Blood studies show Hct 32, WBC 10,000 and a sedimentation rate of 108. The serum creatinine is elevated to 2.1 and the BUN is 30.

John Dory's intravenous pyelogram (Fig. 3) shows that the left kidney is diffusely enlarged and the renal pelvis is compressed.

What are your thoughts at this stage? How will you proceed?

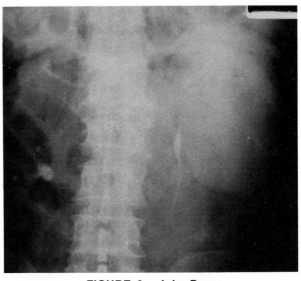

FIGURE 3. John Dory

Your first thought is probably that **John Dory** has an extensive tumor in the left kidney, either a late metastasis from the right renal carcinoma or a second primary tumor. This thought is encouraged by the very high sedimentation rate, a very common feature of renal carcinoma. If the lesion is malignant, the outlook is very gloomy because *Mr. Dory* would not be a very good subject for nephrectomy and cadaver kidney transplantation, but it is sometimes possible to resect a tumor from a solitary kidney and so you request renal angiography to clarify the diagnosis (Figs. 4 and 5).

You can see that there is no evidence of tumor. The outer border of the kidney is flattened. Lateral to the lower two thirds of the kidney there is a less dense shadow with a smooth, convex outer margin. There is extensive disease of the renal artery.

This is a rare condition, spontaneous subcapsular hematoma of the kidney, a sort of renal apoplexy.

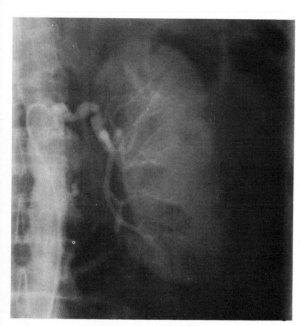

FIGURE 4. John Dory

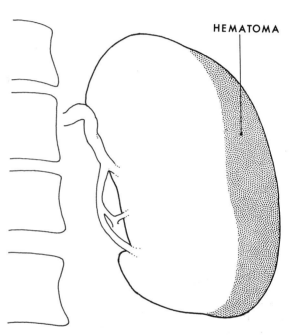

HEMATOMA

FIGURE 5. John Dory

Mr. Dory's diagnosis was confirmed at surgery and the hematoma was evacuated. Material taken for biopsy from the hematoma capsule revealed no carcinoma. Postoperatively, renal function returned to normal, as did the intravenous pyelogram, which you can see in Figure 6.

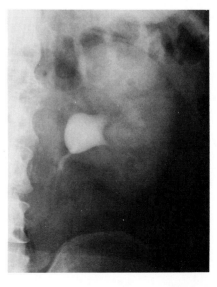

FIGURE 6. John Dory

Pedro Spinoza, a 40 year old Mexican who sells hot dogs at the ball park, complains of an aching pain in his right loin that has been present for the past 6 months. He says that on two or three occasions the pain was quite severe for a few days. You notice that he walks with a limp, and you find that his left hip is fixed, with 7 cm shortening of his left leg. He explains that he was kicked by a mule when he was 7 years old and that his hip became stiff over the next six months. Apart from this, he has always been very healthy, and physical examination discloses no other abnormality. Routine laboratory tests are normal. You request x-ray studies of his hips and lumbar spine and a plain film of the abdomen (Fig. 7). See what you can make of this film before turning to page 6.

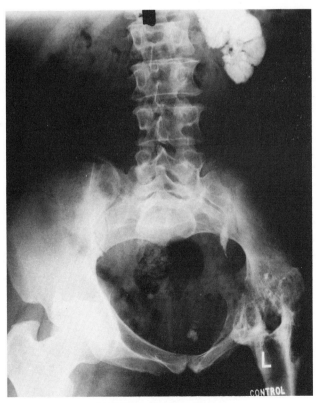

FIGURE 7. Pedro Spinoza

In **Pedro Spinoza's** case there is so much to comment on that it may be difficult to know where to start. It is always a good plan to begin with the bones. You can see why his left hip is fixed. The acetabulum and the head of the left femur have disappeared and there is complete bony ankylosis. This is the final result of untreated tuberculosis of the hip. Did you notice the consequent deformity of the pelvis?

Now look at the large calcified mass in the upper left abdomen. From its shape it is clearly a completely calcified kidney. You can even see the fetal lobulation. Even without the clue from the hip disease you should recognize this as the end stage of renal tuberculosis, sometimes described as an *autonephrectomy*. At the level of the pelvic brim and also at the L5 level there is calcification of the ureter. Above the pubic symphysis you can see calcification of the left seminal vesicle and you should have been able to feel this on rectal examination.

Go back to *Mr. Spinoza* and make a more careful examination of his scrotum. Did you miss something the first time? Yes, the left epididymis is firmly thickened and irregular, again a healed TB lesion, but this time healed by fibrosis rather than calcification.

You may wonder at such extensive disease without any history of illness, but unless there is secondary infection urinary tuberculosis is often silent if the bladder is not involved.

But what has all this to do with *Mr. Spinoza's* complaint of aching pain in the right loin? What about the opacity in the right side of the pelvis about 3½ cm medial to the right ischial spine? Is this another calcified tuberculosis lesion? No; contrast the sharp outline and uniform density with the irregular, mottled appearance of the tuberculosis lesions. This is much more likely to be a stone in the right ureter so you had better look at the IVP.

Pedro Spinoza's IVP (Fig. 8) completes the story. There is of course no sign of excretion from the left kidney. On the right side there is duplication of the renal pelvis and ureter. The lower segment ureter is dilated because it is obstructed by the stone at the lower end and this is the cause of *Mr. Spinoza's* pain.

The stone was removed by open surgery and analysis showed that it was an oxalate stone. Repeated special cultures of the urine for tubercle bacilli are negative and the blood calcium is normal, so *Mr. Spinoza* can return to his hot dog stand without further ado.

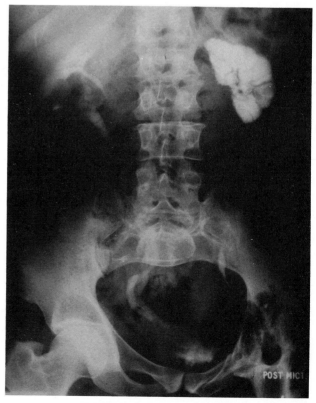

FIGURE 8. Pedro Spinoza

Jay Walker, age 27, an unemployed winebibber, is brought to the emergency room after an unsuccessful attempt to weave his way across a busy street. He had been felled by a cruising taxicab, and a wheel had passed over his abdomen. Apart from the aura of alcohol, the only abnormal feature on clinical examination is acute tenderness in the loin and upper abdomen on the right side. Nothing significant is found in routine x-rays of chest, abdomen and pelvis, but you discover blood in his urine. What additional x-ray studies would you request at this stage and why?

Obviously you suspect injury to **Jay Walker's** right kidney. In all such cases it is essential to obtain an IVP immediately for two reasons: to acquire further information about the damaged kidney and, even more important, to discover the status of the kidney on the other side. If the patient goes into shock and emergency surgery is needed to control hemorrhage, it is vital to know that there is another functioning kidney.

Figure 9 is the 10 minute film from the pyelogram. What do you make of it?

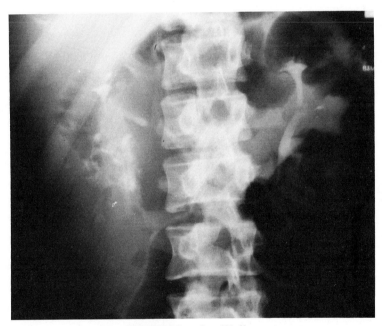

FIGURE 9. Jay Walker

The first point to note is that **Jay Walker's** left kidney is present and functioning well. On the right side the irregular pattern of the contrast medium indicates extravasation. A large mass has displaced the hepatic flexure of the colon. This is a perirenal hematoma. Clearly *Mr. Walker's* right kidney is ruptured. What further studies might be helpful?

As you see, a selective renal angiogram was obtained (Fig. 10). There is a large split in the middle of the kidney, but the renal artery and its main branches are intact. The capsular arteries are not usually visible, but here they are clearly seen because the capsule has been lifted from the parenchyma by subcapsular hematoma.

As long as the capsule remains intact, the pressure of the hematoma tends to control the bleeding from the torn renal tissue. In fact, *Mr. Walker's* vital signs remained stable and he recovered uneventfully without surgery. See below for the end of the story.

Figure 11 is from a selective angiogram study made six months after **Jay Walker's** accident. You can see how the kidney has healed, leaving a large central scar. The IVP at this time was essentially normal.

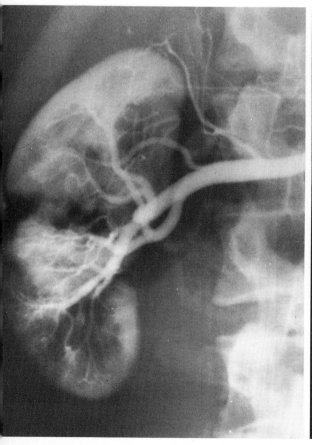

FIGURE 10. Jay Walker

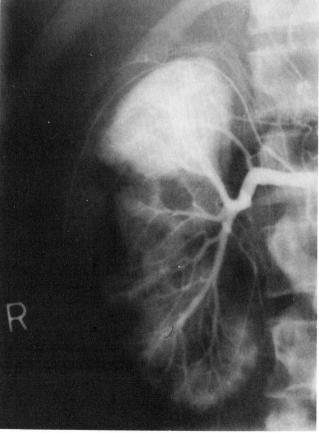

FIGURE 11. Jay Walker

Mary Leaky, age 12, is the pampered daughter of a much married actress, Lulu Bolsover. Lulu complains bitterly that she cannot send *Mary* away to school because she wets her bed. Lulu has tried almost as many psychiatrists as husbands but the problem persists. Neurologic consultation has not been helpful: there is no evidence of any nerve lesion to account for the lack of control.

Urinalysis shows rather more WBCs than normal and culture produces *E. coli* with a colony count of 50,000, which is rather indeterminate.

You request an IVP. Figure 12 is the 10 minute film: it seems normal. Does this imply that Mary's problem is in fact psychological?

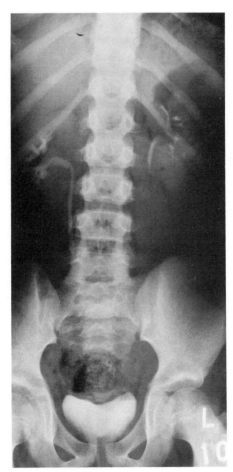

FIGURE 12.   Mary Leaky

No, **Mary Leaky's** normal IVP does not rule out serious urinary disorder. Figure 13 is a spot film taken during micturating cystography. It shows gross vesicoureteral reflux. Incidentally, this film was taken while *Mary* was standing, and it shows considerable ptosis of the right kidney that was not apparent in the IVP.

Both of *Mary's* ureters were reimplanted into her bladder with an anti-reflux procedure and she was given prolonged antibiotic therapy. She gradually became dry at night in the subsequent eight months and Lulu celebrated by getting married again.

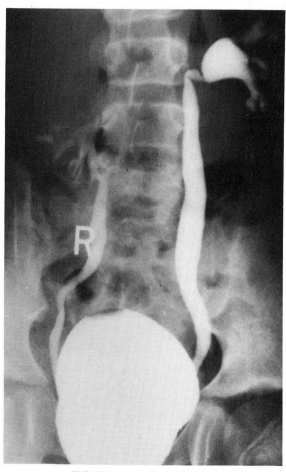

FIGURE 13. Mary Leaky

Dolly Doyle, a 24 year old waitress, complains that during the past year or so she has been subject to attacks of frequent micturition, including a degree of urgency that makes waiting difficult. She has no other symptoms and no history of previous illness.

Complete physical examination and routine lab studies reveal no abnormality. Her urine is normal and sterile.

An IVP has been requested and Figure 14 is the preliminary plain film. What do you make of the opacity to the left of the twelfth thoracic vertebra?

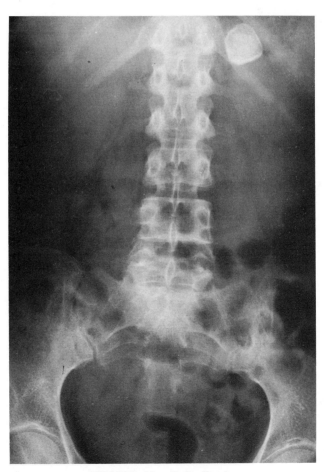

FIGURE 14. Dolly Doyle

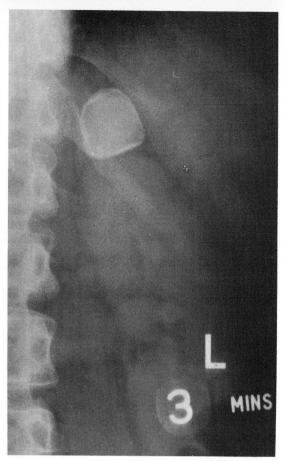

FIGURE 15. Dolly Doyle

The opacity shown in **Dolly Doyle's** IVP is a calcified adrenal gland. Figure 15 is the 3 minute film and Figure 16 a 10 minute oblique film from the IVP series, and they clearly show the relationship of the opacity to the kidney.

The lesion is most likely to be a calcified hematoma. Spontaneous bleeding into the adrenal gland is not rare, especially in infancy.

This chance discovery has little significance. *Dolly's* problem is almost certainly a urethral syndrome, but she should have cystourethroscopy to complete the work-up.

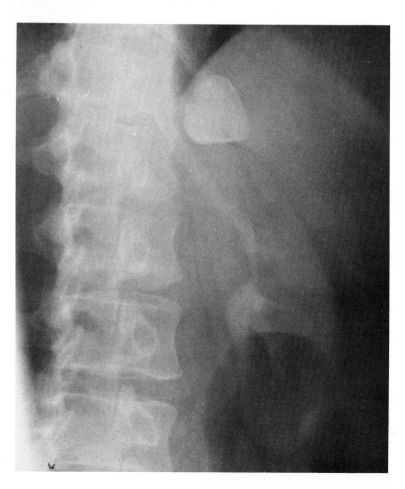

FIGURE 16. Dolly Doyle

Barney Wall, age 35, a prosperous stockbroker, is brought to the emergency room by his wife. An hour earlier he had been smitten by a sudden severe pain in the upper left abdomen that radiated into the left loin and down to the left pubic region. He is very distressed. You elicit tenderness in the left flank and left costovertebral angle.

What do you think is wrong? What immediate studies are indicated?

Barney Wall has a classic renal colic. The essential immediate studies are microscopic examination of the urine and intravenous urography. *Mr. Wall* is likely to have a small stone in his left ureter. He might void the stone in the next few hours, and if you merely prescribe an analgesic and postpone the studies to the following morning you may find every-thing normal and you will be left wondering if your diagnosis was correct.

If severe pain is due to a lesion in the urinary tract, there is nearly always a significant number of red cells in a *relevant urine;* that is, urine that has been voided while the pain was still present.

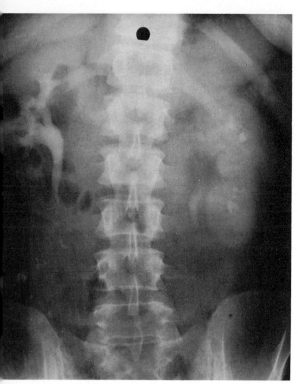

FIGURE 17. Barney Wall

Barney Wall's urine contains a large number of red cells. No calculus is visible in the preliminary film. On the 20 minute film (Fig. 17), it can be seen that the left ureter is obstructed at the L3 level. There is a dense nephrogram and as yet the pelvis and calyces are incompletely filled with contrast medium.

The stone was passed spontaneously four days later. Fortunately, it was retrieved and proved to consist of uric acid. This is important because it ought to be possible to prevent further stone production by appropriate medical management.

The opacities seen below the right kidney are old, calcified mesenteric lymph nodes.

Are you satisfied with the appearance of the right upper tract?

There is slight obstruction of the right ureter at the level of the L2–L3 interspace. This was overlooked at the time but became visible through the retrospectoscope a year later, when *Mr. Wall* complained of mild lumbar backache and another IVP was performed.

On the 5 minute film (Fig. 18), the left kidney is normal but on the right side the obstruction of the upper ureter is obvious.

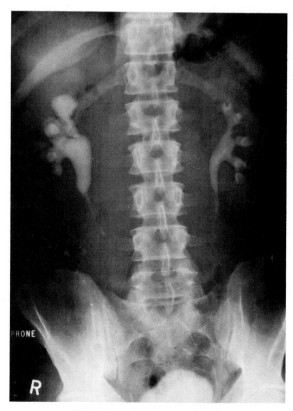

FIGURE 18. Barney Wall

It was not really necessary, but the obstruction was confirmed after taking the 15 minute film by injecting 40 mg of frusemide and taking another film 10 minutes later (Fig. 19). The fast acting diuretic has largely washed out the contrast medium on the left but there has been no washout on the right.

The upper ureteral region on the right was explored surgically and the obstruction was found to be caused by a very extensive retroperitoneal mass.

Biopsy of the mass revealed Hodgkin's disease. This was treated by a combination of radiotherapy and cytotoxic drugs.

Figure 20 is a combined lymphogram and IVP. You can see considerably enlarged glands at the pelvic brim and along both iliac chains, but above the L5 level the contrast medium has spread out into a great network corresponding to the large retroperitoneal mass of Hodgkin tissue.

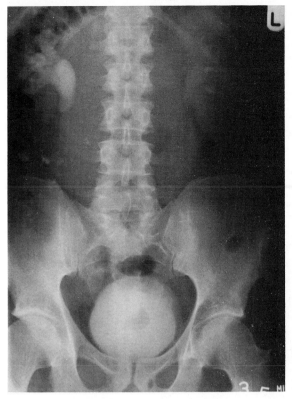

FIGURE 19. Barney Wall

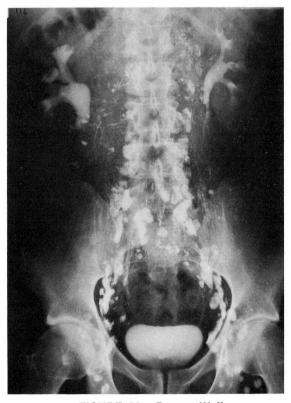

FIGURE 20. Barney Wall

Hank Mooney, 27, a traffic cop, is referred by his family doctor because of recurrent attacks of epididymitis and urinary infection. He brings IVP films with him. Figure 21 is the preliminary film and Figure 22 is the 10 minute film. What do you make of them?

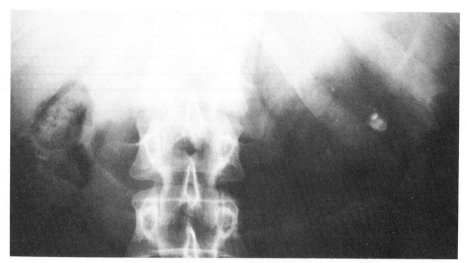

FIGURE 21. Hank Mooney

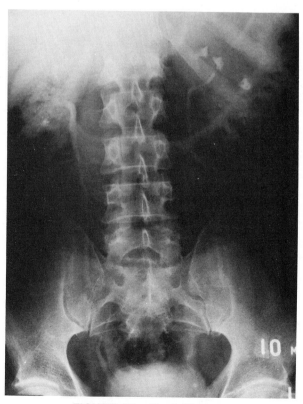

FIGURE 22. Hank Mooney

Hank Mooney's films are not good but you can see what appear to be stones scattered through the calyces of both kidneys. On the right side much of the detail is obscured by feces in the colon, but there is no gross abnormality in the pyelogram. The left side is rather curious.

There is no renal pelvis as such: the ureter runs directly to the upper calyces and no contrast medium is visible in the lower two thirds of the left kidney.

Do you think there is a space occupying lesion in the lower part of the left kidney?

Before giving an opinion on **Hank Mooney,** you had better have a look at the film taken after voiding (Fig. 23). This gives a lot of new information that was not apparent in the earlier films of the series. There is duplication of the entire upper tract on the left with hydronephrosis of the lower segment and considerable dilatation of the lower segment ureter. The upper segment ureter is a little dilated in comparison with the earlier films. Immediately above the left ischial spine, outside the line of the ureter, there is a phlebolith.

What do you think now? Would any other x-ray studies be helpful?

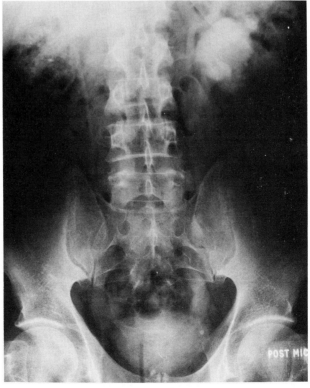

FIGURE 23. Hank Mooney

The only logical explanation for the urographic appearances is reflux up *both left ureters*. The next step is to request a voiding cystogram. Two of the spot films are shown in Figures 24 and 25. Figure 24 is a resting film showing gross reflux up both ureters. Figure 25 is a film taken during voiding, and now you can see gross distention of the lower segment renal pelvis which has totally destroyed the lower part of *Mr. Mooney's* kidney.

The useless lower segment will be removed together with its entire ureter; if a stump of this ureter were left, it would act as a bladder diverticulum and perpetuate infection.

At a later stage, the upper segment ureter will be reimplanted into the bladder, using an anti-reflux procedure. *Hank* should then be able to return happily to giving out tickets, but his stones will have to be watched.

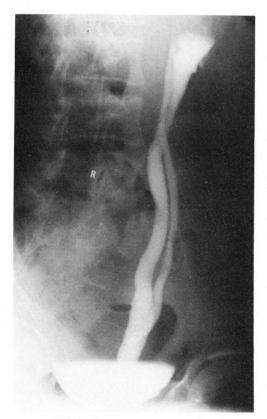

FIGURE 24. Hank Mooney

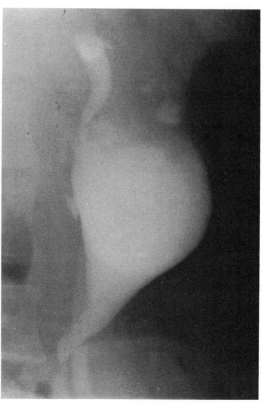

FIGURE 25. Hank Mooney

Babs Rikker, age 20, is a telephone operator. In childhood she was totally incontinent of urine, because of "something missing in the lower part of her spine." When she was five, her urine was diverted to her abdominal wall by an ileal conduit. She has had no problems with this and she is able to manage her collecting appliance very well.

In recent months *Babs* has not been feeling well, has had repeated chills, and has noticed that her urine is often muddy.

Spina bifida is the commonest cause of neuropathic bladder requiring urinary diversion in childhood, but you find no sign of this on physical examination. Urine culture gives a heavy growth of *Proteus*. Figure 26 is her plain film.

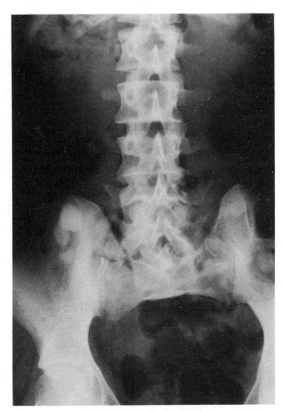

FIGURE 26. Babs Rikker

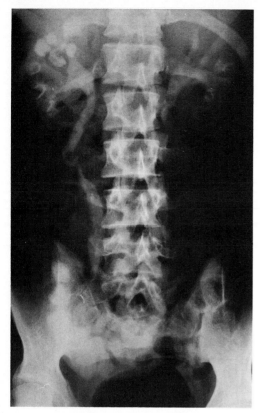

FIGURE 27. Babs Rikker

Babs Rikker is not afflicted with spina bifida, but did you observe the absence of the lower part of the sacrum. The partial agenesis of the sacrum was the cause of the cauda equina lesion responsible for the bladder malfunction. There are three large opacities on the right side at the L5 level. You suspect that these may be stones in the ileal conduit and you request an IVP. Figure 27 is the 25 minute film.

Yes, there are three stones in the conduit. **Babs Rikker's** left kidney seems normal but there is some dilatation of the whole upper tract on the right side. This might be due to mild stenosis of the anastomosis of the right ureter with the ileal loop, so you request a loopogram (Fig. 28). This shows the stones as filling defects and there is free reflux up both ureters, as there should be, proving that there is no stricture.

The reason for the stone formation is stasis in the conduit due to contraction of the stoma. The loopogram shows that the loop is too long. Even if a conduit is properly made as short as possible, it tends to elongate with passage of time. An ileal conduit is one of the best methods of urinary diversion but no method is perfect, and after 12 to 15 years ileal chickens begin to come home to roost.

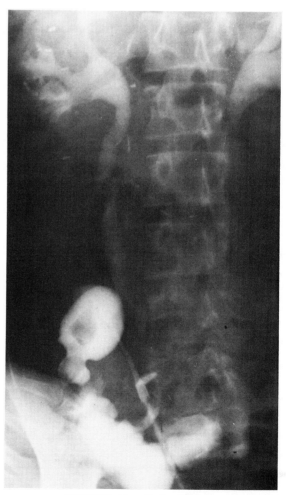

FIGURE 28. Babs Rikker

Bertie Bloop, a 28 year old house painter, is referred to your clinic for urologic investigation because he has to pass urine every hour during the day. He has had some degree of frequency as long as he can remember but it had got worse recently. Further questioning elicits the information that he cannot micturate in company and that he has a non-competitive stream. Physical examination and routine lab studies are normal. His urine is normal and sterile. Turn to page 22 for *Bertie's* intravenous urogram.

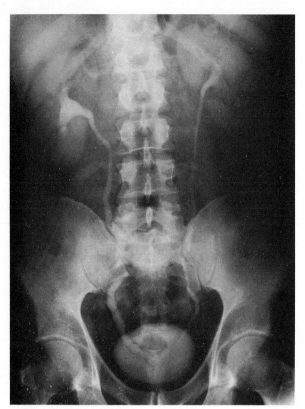

FIGURE 29.   Bertie Bloop

Figure 29 is the 10 minute film. **Bertie Bloop's** kidneys are normal. The right ureter is a little dilated. Both ureters are somewhat tortuous, and both can be seen in their entire length. You do not normally see the whole ureter on one film and, if you do, it suggests obstruction at the lower end.

Within the cystogram (Fig. 30) is the characteristic cobra-head outline of a ureterocele on the right side. If you look very closely, you may be able to discern a tiny ureterocele on the left side also. This is a chance discovery, entirely unrelated to *Bertie's* problem, which is a hyperactive bladder.

There is a clue to this diagnosis in the appearance of the bladder, which is very rounded at a relatively small volume, with a thick bladder wall.

The ureteroceles will probably be slit or unroofed transurethrally to relieve obstruction. Urodynamic studies are indicated for further evaluation of the bladder problem.

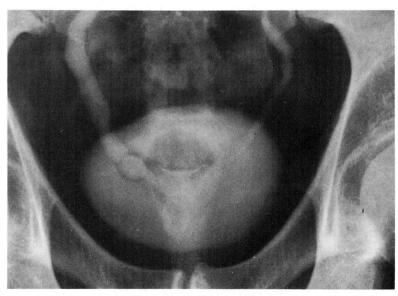

FIGURE 30.   Bertie Bloop

Hans Dietl, age 25, used-car salesman, passed blood-stained urine late last night after a long session on the beer with a prospective customer. He is very scared. His urine this morning looks clear but on microscopy is found to contain many red cells. This is of some importance, to confirm that the red color that frightened him was in fact caused by blood. Figure 31 is the 30 minute film from his IVP (the preliminary film was normal).

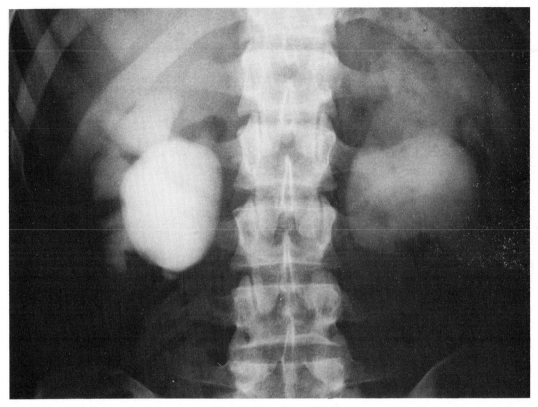

FIGURE 31. Hans Dietl

Hans Dietl has a moderately severe, bilateral hydronephrosis, almost certainly congenital, caused by partial obstruction at the ureteropelvic junction.

It is curious how advanced hydronephrosis may be without producing symptoms, and it is also difficult to see why hematuria should occur, as in the present case. The hematuria may be associated with the distention caused by the beer diuresis. The effect of diuresis is shown dramatically by giving 40 mg of frusemide at this stage of the IVP. For the result, please turn to page 24.

Figure 32 is the film taken five minutes after injecting frusemide. It confirms that the obstruction on each side is in fact at the ureteropelvic junction and not lower down. This is a helpful trick in cases where there is some doubt about the presence of obstruction, as may happen if the patient is underhydrated at the time of the IVP. Don't forget to give the patient plenty to drink when you inject the diuretic, or you may produce acute dehydration.

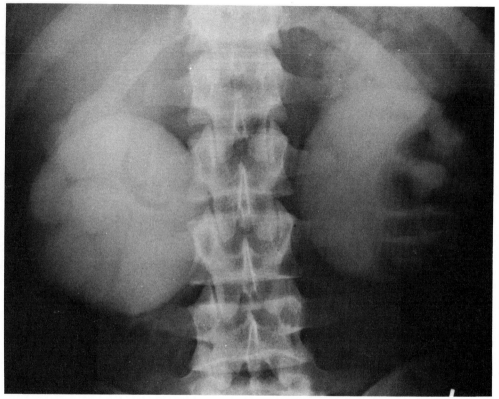

FIGURE 32. Hans Dietl

You must first cystoscope **Hans Dietl** to be sure that the bleeding did not come from a papillary bladder tumor. If the bladder is normal you can carry on with pyeloplasty, doing one side at a time.

Hoppy Alcatraz, age 65, is a short-tempered ex-convict. He presents himself in the Emergency Room late on Saturday night demanding "a shot of penicillin to fix the kidneys." Although he is not an easy conversationalist, you manage to discover that he has had severe frequency and burning micturition since early morning. Urinalysis shows 2+ albumin with a sediment containing a large number of WBCs and some RBCs.

Do you accept his diagnosis of urinary infection and prescribe an antibiotic?

If **Hoppy Alcatraz** has a urinary infection, it has not appeared without a predisposing cause, and further study is indicated. Even more important is the fact that acute cystitis in older people may not be caused by infection: It is essential to have a clean-catch specimen of urine for culture before starting an antibiotic (although you do not need to wait for the result).

In fact, *Hoppy's* urine is sterile. His IVP is shown below.

There is a big filling defect in *Hoppy Alcatraz's* bladder. What will you do now?

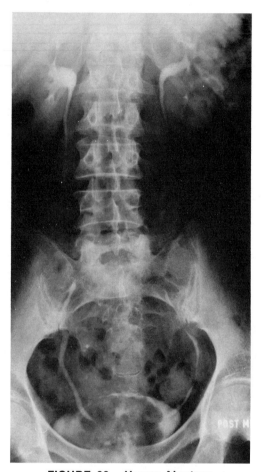

FIGURE 33. Hoppy Alcatraz

The filling defect in **Hoppy Alcatraz's** bladder is a large carcinoma. The next step is cystoscopy and bimanual palpation under anesthesia to determine the stage of the tumor. During cystoscopy, adequate material must be resected from the tumor for full histologic assessment and grading. All this information is necessary before you can make any decision about treatment.

Godiva Catchpenny was famous in her youth for her equestrian exploits but now, at the age of 81, she is more notable for the dazzling brilliance of her war paint. Her family doctor has referred her because he is worried about her recurrent urinary infections and backache. You request an IVP.

No calculi were seen in **Ms. Catchpenny's** preliminary film. The IVP (Fig. 34) shows a moderately large hydronephrosis on the left. The picture on the right is more sinister. The pelvis and calyces are deformed and displaced by a large space-occupying lesion. Will you request renal arteriography?

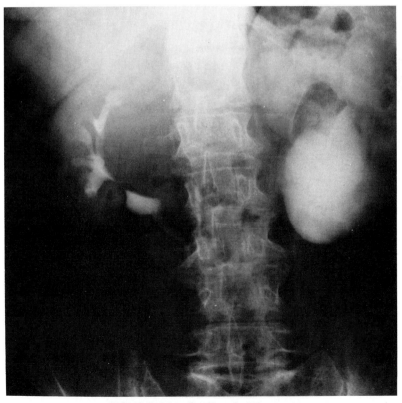

FIGURE 34. Godiva Catchpenny

Renal arteriography is not to be undertaken lightly in **Godiva,** a lady of 81 winters. Your object is to find out if the mass in the right kidney is a malignant tumor or a harmless cyst. The smooth, circular outline of the lesion strongly suggests a cyst, and it may be possible to confirm the diagnosis with much less risk.

Under radiographic control, using an image intensifier and television monitor, a long needle was passed into the lesion in **Godiva Catchpenny's** kidney. Clear fluid was withdrawn and sent for cytology, and then contrast medium was injected. The spot film (Fig. 35) shows a large parapelvic cyst.

Surgery is not indicated for either kidney. *Ms. Catchpenny's* back pain is caused by the severe osteoarthritis of her spine. Her urinary infection is secondary to senile atrophic stenosis of her external urethral meatus, which can be treated simply by meatotomy and urethral dilatation, together with appropriate urinary antiseptics.

By the way, when you are explaining the condition to the Lady Godiva, do not use the word senile if you value her custom!

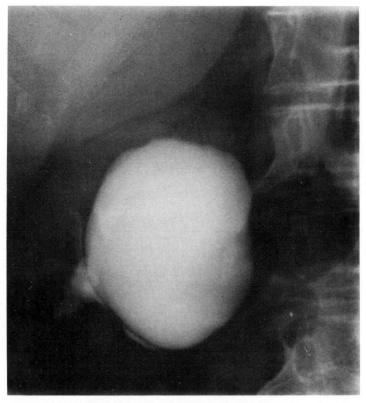

FIGURE 35. Godiva Catchpenny

Ethel Reddy, age 24, works as a stenographer. She complains of severe pain in the left flank radiating to the lower left quadrant of the abdomen. She says that she has had a similar pain on several previous occasions in the past couple of years, but she is rather vague about it. Urine and stat blood studies are normal. You request a plain film of the abdomen.

Ethel Reddy's plain film (Fig. 36) shows a small opacity on the left side between the transverse processes of L3 and L4. It lies in the line of the left ureter. Do you think it is a ureteral stone?

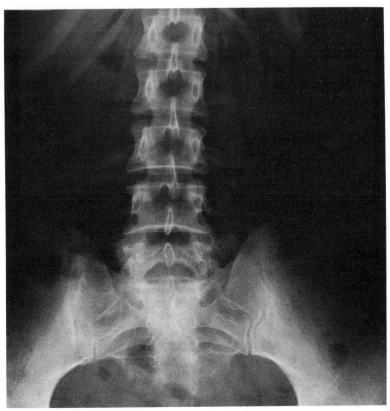

FIGURE 36. Ethel Reddy

An IVP (Fig. 37) shows that the opacity lies outside **Ethel's** left ureter and that it has moved up just above the transverse process of L3. It is probably a small, calcified mesenteric gland.

Careful enquiry elicits the fact that *Ethel's* pain began on the fourteenth day of her menstrual cycle. She is slim, and it is not difficult to reach her ovaries on rectal examination. The left ovary is distinctly tender.

Miss Reddy's pain is a *Mittelschmerz*, or ovulation pain. You prescribe some simple analgesic and ask her to note carefully the relationship of any future attacks to her menstrual cycle.

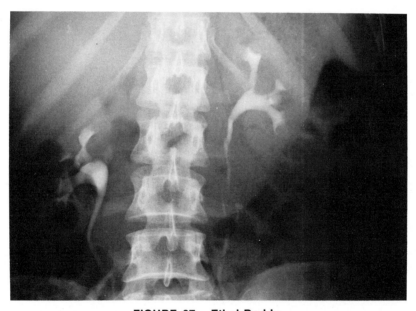

FIGURE 37. Ethel Reddy

Chet Murphy, age 27, a professional golfer, has been transferred to your hospital for treatment of acute renal failure that followed an automobile accident. His only serious injuries were multiple compound fractures of the left leg but he lost a great deal of blood and the leg had to be amputated.

For seven weeks after the accident he produced very little urine, not more than 10 or 20 ml per day, and he was maintained on frequent hemodialysis. Then, very slowly, the urinary output increased and he has not needed dialysis for the past two weeks; however, it is now 15 weeks since the accident and his serum creatinine is falling very gradually: it is now 8. What are your thoughts about the case at this stage?

Chet Murphy's is no ordinary case of acute tubular necrosis. The oliguric phase of acute tubular necrosis rarely lasts more than three or four weeks at most and, once diuresis returns, recovery is usually much faster. You suspect that there is some other problem, perhaps a kidney disease antedating the accident. Renal biopsy is indicated but, before doing this, is there any other study that might be helpful?

A high-dose nephrotomogram was obtained (Fig. 38). **Chet's** kidneys are small. Each kidney is outlined by a thin rim of calcification, seen better on the left side, but visible on both sides on the original film. *Chet* has bilateral cortical necrosis. The diagnosis was confirmed by renal biopsy.

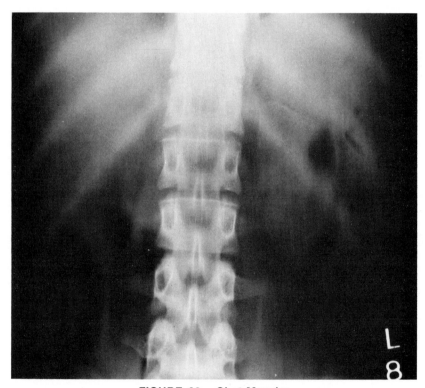

FIGURE 38.   Chet Murphy

Cortical necrosis is usually found only as a complication of toxemic ante-partum hemorrhage and it is rare in men. In **Chet Murphy's** case it must be patchy and incomplete, otherwise there would be no renal function at all.

Chet's serum creatinine finally lev-elled out at 3.5 and at that stage an IVP (Fig. 39) looked surprisingly good.

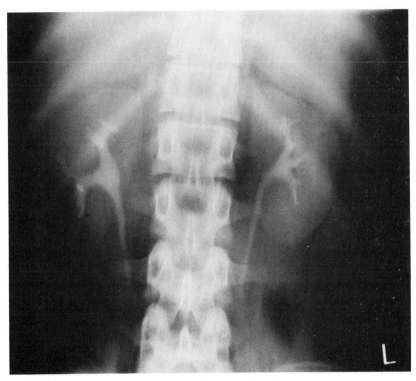

FIGURE 39.   Chet Murphy

Sarah Fine, age 42, is brought by her husband, an internist, because she passed blood clots in her urine a few hours earlier. Apart from a strikingly high facial color, physical examination is unremarkable. Urinalysis confirms the presence of blood. Hematocrit is 52, and the corrected sedimentation rate is 120. What is your diagnosis and how would you confirm it?

Isolated hematuria—that is, hematuria with no other symptom—is considered to be caused by tumor in the urinary tract or kidney until proved otherwise. The very high sedimentation rate revealed in **Sarah** is common in renal carcinoma, and the polycythemia is also extremely suggestive. The kidney has several endocrine functions, including production of erythropoietin, so it is not surprising to find polycythemia in some patients with renal carcinoma. See page 35 for *Mrs. Fine's* intravenous pyelogram.

This 10 minute film from **Sarah Fine's** IVP (Fig. 40) has many interesting features. What are your comments?

On the right side there is one large and many small gallstones, with a rim of calcification around lucent centers. These were, of course, seen in the preliminary film. **Sarah's** right kidney is normal. On the left side, the renal pelvis and lower calyces are filled with clot outlined by a thin film of contrast medium. The upper and middle calyces are missing, and the upper border of the pelvis is indented by a space-occupying lesion. Will you now proceed with surgery?

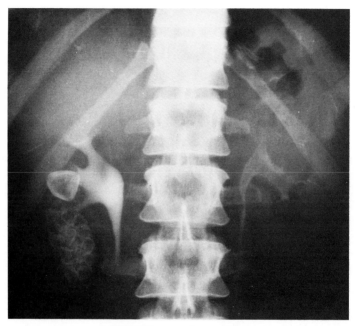

FIGURE 40.   Sarah Fine

You should first request selective renal arteriograms on **Sarah** to get more information about the tumor. The arterial phase (Fig. 41) shows the classical mottled confusion of the vessels, and the nephrogram phase (Fig. 42) shows that the tumor is well defined, with no apparent extension beyond the kidney capsule, and so, provided that there are no metastases, the prognosis may be good.

Ordinary nephrectomy will not do. It is essential to do a radical nephrectomy for the best chance of cure. The renal artery and vein must be secured before any handling of the kidney to minimize the risk of tumor embolism from this very vascular carcinoma during surgery. This is one tumor in which the technical skill of the operator really does affect the prognosis.

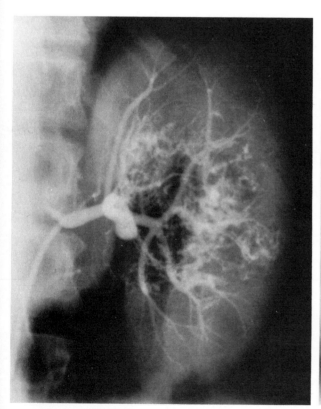

FIGURE 41. Sarah Fine

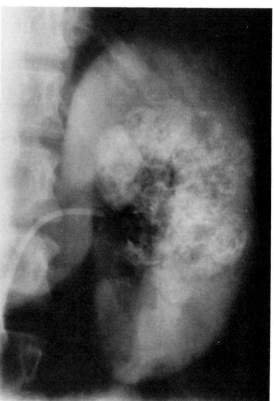

FIGURE 42. Sarah Fine

Betty Hely, age about 60, is one of the derelicts of modern urban life. She was picked off the sidewalk by the police, who found her propped against the wall, mumbling and incoherent. She was first thought to be drunk but her breath, though foul, was innocent of alcohol. Your first thought is that she may be diabetic and you arrange stat urine and blood studies while you make a physical examination.

Her blood pressure is 110/60. There is no sign of congestive cardiac failure. There is gross edema of both legs and her abdomen is swollen, and you suspect that it is full of fluid. The nurse who has passed a catheter reports that there is no urine in the bladder. The initial hemogram shows Hct 21, WBC 7000 with 54 polys, 42 lymphocytes and 4 monocytes. The blood glucose is 70, but the BUN is 210 and there is severe acidosis. How will you proceed?

Obviously, **Betty Hely** is uremic, but at this stage you cannot tell whether the renal failure is terminal chronic or acute and reversible. The first step is to institute dialysis to gain time for definitive diagnosis, although the severe anemia suggests that the renal failure is chronic. A plain film shows no calculi, and you cannot see the renal outlines. What will you do now?

The complete anuria points very strongly to post-renal obstruction affecting either both kidneys or a solitary kidney so you do a cystoscopy. Pelvic examination of **Ms. Hely** at the same time reveals no tumor. The bladder is normal, and catheters pass easily to both kidneys. Does this mean that there is no obstruction?

Free passage of ureteral catheters does not rule out obstruction, as you can see when you look at **Betty Hely's** retrograde pyelogram (Fig. 43). There is bilateral hydronephrosis, with the calyces more affected than the pelves. The medial deviation of both ureters indicates retroperitoneal fibrosis. This condition usually spares the great vessels, but here the edema suggests obstruction of the inferior vena cava. How will you confirm this?

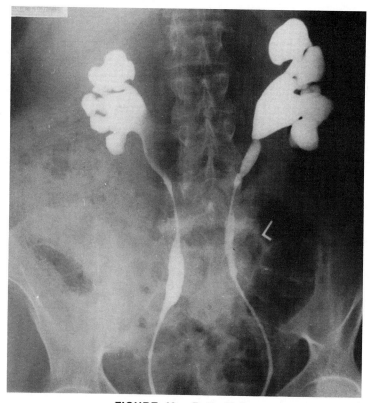

FIGURE 43. Betty Hely

A catheter was inserted into **Betty Hely's** right femoral vein and passed up to the common iliac under fluoroscopic control. After injection of contrast medium, spot films were taken (Figs. 44 and 45). These show complete occlusion of the vena cava and a collateral circulation. Spot films of the left thigh (Fig. 46, shown on page 40) show that clot has propagated all the way down the left femoral vein.

Two days later, pulmonary embolus wrote finis to a sad life. Autopsy confirmed the diagnosis of idiopathic retroperitoneal fibrosis.

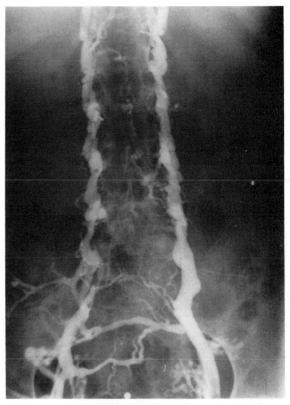

FIGURE 44. Betty Hely

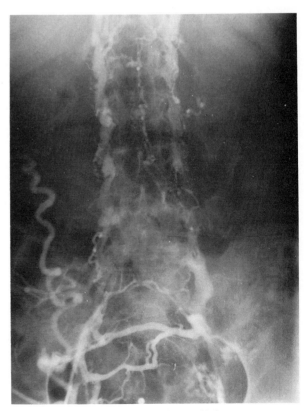

FIGURE 45. Betty Hely

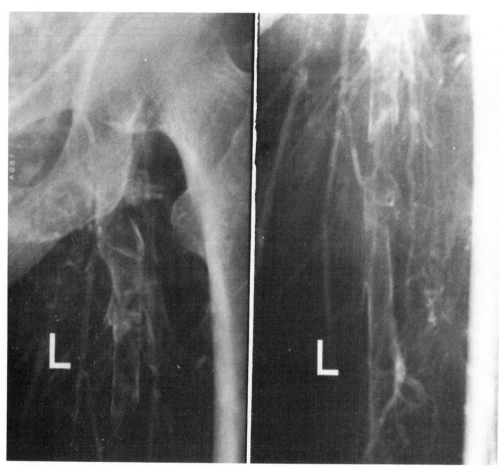

FIGURE 46.   Betty Hely

John Jones, a 42 year old tool polisher, has been having recurrent attacks of lower urinary tract infection for the past year. He comes to your clinic, bringing an intravenous urogram done elsewhere. The films are not good but you are satisfied that they show no abnormality in the upper urinary tract. You decide to outrule vesicoureteral reflux and request micturating cystography. Figure 47 is the spot film taken with the bladder full. Is there reflux into the right ureter?

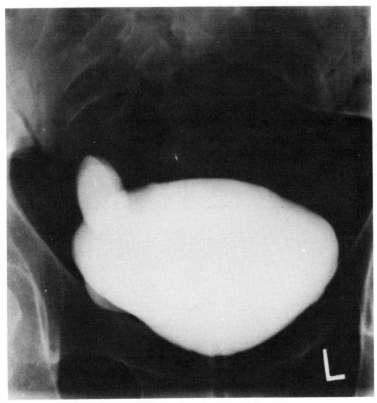

FIGURE 47. John Jones

The projection from the upper right part of **John Jones'** bladder is a diverticulum. Look at the spot film taken during micturition (Fig. 48). You can see how the diverticulum is blown up during voiding and you can also see another, small, diverticulum on the left side. What will you do now?

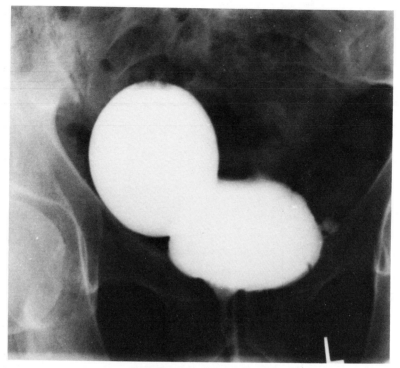

FIGURE 48. **John Jones**

The large diverticulum must be removed: Not only is it a reservoir of infection but also there is a higher incidence of carcinoma in diverticula than in normal bladders. At the same time the cause of the diverticula must be removed. **John Jones** has median bar obstruction at his bladder neck, and this will be relieved, either by transurethral resection or by YV-plasty.

Mike Klunz, a 76 year old retired steelworker, comes to the clinic complaining that "the water doesn't come right." He tells you that he had a gastrectomy 30 years ago and a prostatectomy five years ago. He also suffers from bad arthritis in his right hip. He says that his micturition was never really right after the prostatectomy but it has got much worse in the last six months. On rectal examination you find a slightly enlarged, stony-hard prostate. The urine contains some red and white cells and grows *E. coli* on culture. The hemogram, electrolytes and BUN are normal. The acid and alkaline phosphatases are also normal, but nevertheless you suspect that *Mr. Klunz* has developed carcinoma of the prostate, arising in the capsule, or perhaps present at the time of his prostatectomy five years ago. The histology from that operation is not available. Do you now proceed with prostatic biopsy?

You should first request a plain film (Fig. 49). You can see that someone has forgotten to remove the corset that **Mr. Klunz** wears to control the large incisional hernia in his upper abdomen, and you also note severe arthritic changes in the right hip.

What do you make of the curious opacity in the midline at the level of the pubis?

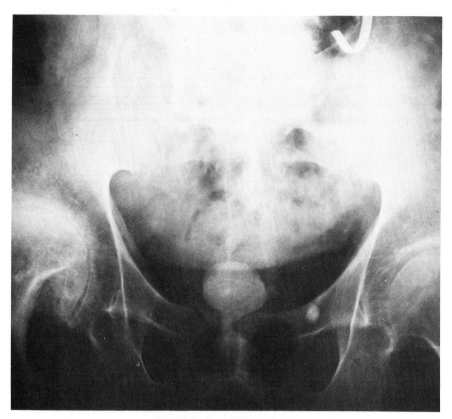

FIGURE 49. Mike Klunz

This is a dumbbell stone. The lower part is in the prostatic cavity, presumably it developed on a devitalized tag of tissue left at the time of **Mr. Klunz's** prostatectomy. It has grown up through the bladder neck, and the upper part is mushrooming into the bladder.

The smaller opacity to the left of the stone is a large phlebolith.

The offending concretion was removed through an incision into the bladder and *Mr. Klunz* was delighted with the restoration of normal micturition.

Thirty year old **Eulalia Gloop** complains of an aching pain in her back, about L3 level. It is particularly bad early in the morning. Physical examination and blood and urine studies are normal. A plain film and x-rays of the lumbar spine reveal no abnormality. You decide to request intravenous urography and, while you are studying the films (Fig. 50), a passing medical student comments on the absence of the right kidney. Do you congratulate him on his perspicacity? Please turn to page 46.

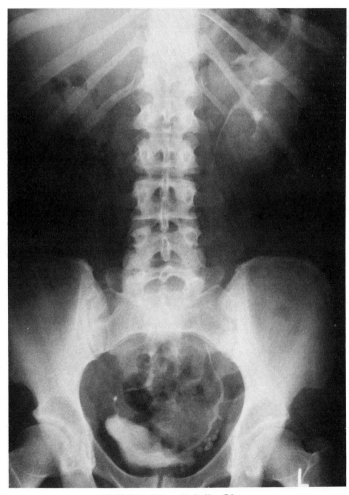

FIGURE 50. Eulalia Gloop

Whenever a kidney is not seen in its normal position, you should search for an ectopic kidney. This may be quite difficult to spot if it lies over dense bone but in the present case it is easy to follow the right ureter up from the bladder to the pelvic kidney.

Eulalia Gloop's backache will probably be relieved by getting her to sleep with boards under her mattress.

Theophrastus Such (you will find his name on all the best police blotters from coast to coast),* a 60 year old reprobate, has been less than fastidious in a half century of venery and, by way of souvenirs, he has acquired a fine collection of urethral strictures. He has had chronic urinary infection for decades and somewhere along the line he lost his right kidney; he is not sure why.

Figure 51 shows part of two of the films of the left kidney and ureter from an IVP series. What do you make of these films?

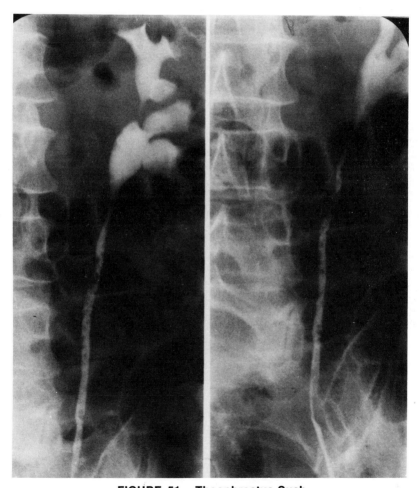

FIGURE 51. Theophrastus Such

Winterset by Maxwell Anderson — Act II:
"My name?
"Theophrastus Such. That's respectable.
"You'll find it all the way from here to the coast on the best police blotters."

As you see, there is a large number of small, round filling defects in the left ureter of **Theophrastus Such.** In the original film, similar filling defects are visible in the renal pelvis and major calyces; you may just be able to spot them in the prints reproduced here.

This is a typical picture of pyelo-ureteritis cystica, usually associated with basal cystitis cystica. This is a curious and not very common disease that develops in people with chronic urinary infection. Its interest is not so much practical as academic.

Lily Bolero, age 51, wife of the Carthaginian consul, is being investigated by a colleague. He has to leave town unexpectedly and asks you to take over the case. He tells you that *Mrs. Bolero* had gross hematuria for one day, and that so far the only significant finding is that the IVP shows a normal left upper tract but no trace of any function on the right side. He has requested right renal angiography.

Figure 52 is the early arterial phase and Figure 53 is the nephrogram phase of **Lily Bolero's** angiographic study. What is your diagnosis?

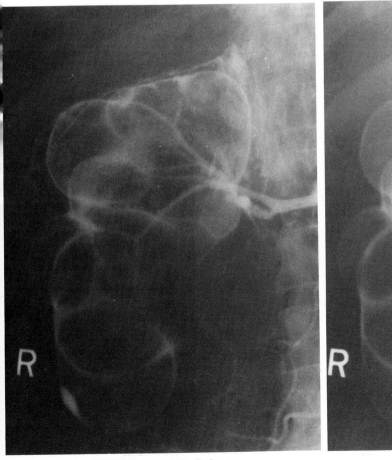

FIGURE 52. Lily Bolero

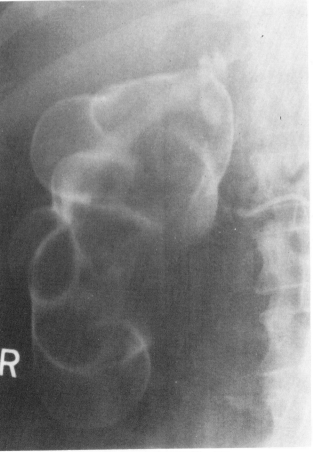

FIGURE 53. Lily Bolero

Lily Bolero's right kidney is a hydronephrotic shell, totally destroyed and presumably the end stage of congenital hydronephrosis. Is any other investigation indicated? Would you have conducted the study in the same way?

The hydronephrosis is quite irrelevant. Cystoscopy disclosed a papillary carcinoma in the bladder, and this was the source of Mrs. Bolero's hematuria.

When a kidney is not visualized on intravenous urography, the next step in investigation should be the simple procedure of cystoscopy, ureteral catheterization and retrograde pyelography. To proceed instead to renal angiography is an abuse of sophisticated technique that is by no means free from risk, even though it may produce pretty pictures.

Forty-seven-year-old **Millie Malaprop** has been in the hospital for a few days, being investigated for post-menopausal vaginal bleeding. Apparently she noticed blood-staining of her underclothes on a few occasions in recent weeks. Your gynecological colleague has found no lesion in the pelvic organs to account for *Mrs. Malaprop's* bleeding, and he has requested urologic consultation. Urinalysis reveals protein +2 and the sediment contains red cells. Figure 54 is the plain film.

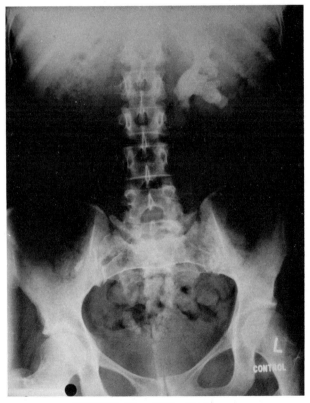

FIGURE 54. Millie Malaprop

You notice the big staghorn calculus in **Millie Malaprop's** left kidney and, incidentally, the heavy fecal loading. Figure 55 is the 60 minute film from the IVP series. What do you make of it?

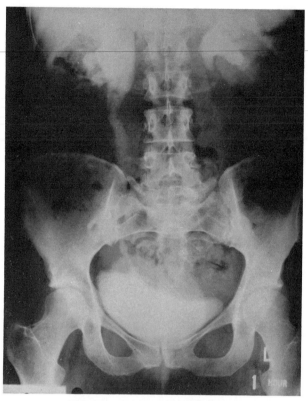

FIGURE 55. Millie Malaprop

There is obviously considerable hydronephrosis and hydroureter on the right side, in addition to the stone in **Millie's** left kidney. Where is the obstruction of the right ureter?

To get a clear view of the obstruction in **Millie Malaprop's** lower ureter, you must look at the film taken after voiding (Fig. 56). There is a large stone in the right ureter at the level of the ischial spine. It is obscured by the bladder in the earlier films. It is in fact visible in the plain film, but camouflaged by the fecal masses.

You must do cystoscopy to rule out bladder neoplasm, but the blood is very likely to have come from one or other upper urinary tract. It is not rare for patients to mistake urinary for vaginal bleeding, and vice versa. *Mrs. Malaprop is not the first person to get things back to front.*

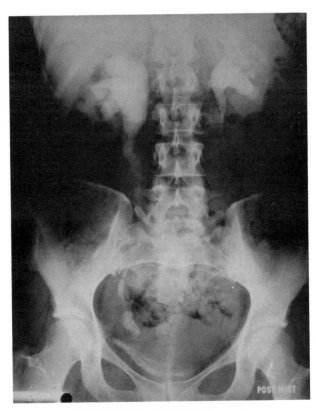

FIGURE 56. Millie Malaprop

Jane Poole, age 24, an airline stewardess, has had incontinence of urine day and night since she was 10 or 11 years old. When a pretty girl in her twenties comes with such a story you can be sure that through the years she has seen many doctors with little success, and you can also be sure that imminent matrimony is the reason that she has decided to make one more effort to be rid of her secret incubus. *Jane* is no exception.

How do you propose to tackle her problem?

All good medicine starts with a careful clinical history. In a case of urinary incontinence this means trying to get a very clear picture of the patient's voiding pattern, and the pattern of the leak. This is not always easy but **Jane Poole** is an intelligent girl, and you discover that she seems to micturate absolutely normally, with no unusual frequency or urgency. Nonetheless, her panties are always wet and she has to wear a pad day and night. The leak does not appear to be associated with effort, and on physical examination you confirm that there is no leak when she coughs with a full bladder.

Jane tells you that a previous cystoscopy in another clinic revealed a normal bladder with normal ureteral orifices.

Do you think that you can solve *Jane's* problem? What will you do?

Jane Poole's condition is very suggestive of ectopic ureter. This would imply duplication of the upper urinary tract on one or both sides, with one or both upper segment ureters opening ectopically somewhere below the level of the external urethral sphincter — perhaps in the vulva or even in the vagina or uterine cervix.

You request an IVP (Fig. 57). There is no apparent duplication. In some cases, the upper segment of a duplex system is so small and so poorly functioning that it does not concentrate the contrast medium, but even then there may be a clue in that the upper segment displaces the upper calyx of the lower segment laterally to give the classic drooping flower appearance, but in this case the pyelogram seems absolutely normal. What do you suggest at this stage?

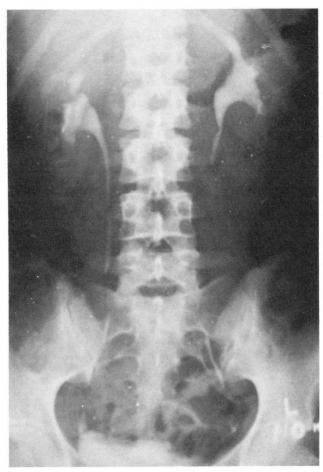

FIGURE 57. Jane Poole

Ten ml of indigo carmine, a deep-blue dye, was instilled into **Jane Poole's** bladder with care to avoid staining the vulva. Three hours later her pad was examined. It was soaking wet but there was no trace of the blue dye. This was the final proof that the leak did not come from the bladder.

The next step was to place *Jane* in the lithotomy position and maintain a continuous watch on the vulval region. After 15 minutes, a jet of clear fluid was seen to spurt from a minute opening 1 cm to the left of the external urethral meatus. A 3F ureteral catheter was inserted into this opening but it would pass only 2 cm. Contrast medium was then injected through the catheter. Much of it leaked back but a spot film (Fig. 58) revealed the lower end of the ectopic ureter passing up on the left side of the pelvis.

At this stage, another ureteral catheter was passed up the normal lower segment ureter. More contrast medium was injected into the ectopic ureter, and in Figure 59 the two ureters can be seen clearly. The contrast medium in the ectopic ureter has passed up to outline faintly a very small upper segment of the left kidney lying just lateral to the space between the twelfth thoracic and first lumbar vertebrae.

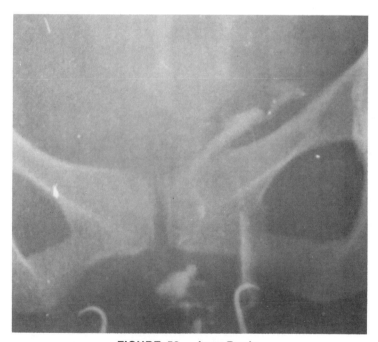

FIGURE 58. Jane Poole

This film shows another common feature of such cases. The lower end of the ectopic ureter is grossly dilated. Use can be made of this fact in eliciting another physical sign — a jet of urine from the ectopic orifice on coughing.

The offending upper segment of the left kidney was removed, and *Jane* became perfectly dry.

Why did she first become wet at the age of 10 or 11? This is a mystery, but there are many well documented cases of girls with an ectopic ureter who did not become wet until about the time of the onset of puberty.

In one respect, *Jane* was lucky. Despite her embarrassing disability, she was a happy girl with a well balanced personality. All too often, failure to diagnose and cure ectopic ureter until the third decade leaves the unfortunate patient a psychosexual cripple.

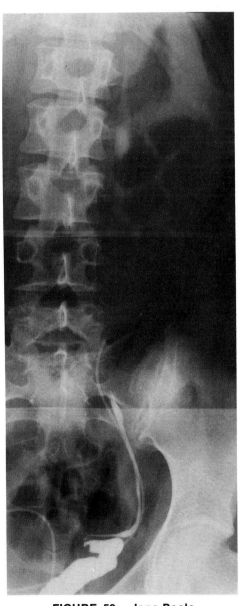

FIGURE 59. Jane Poole

Two years ago, **Carol Owen,** age 27, was found to have end stage renal failure due to bilateral chronic pyelonephritis. After a year on regular dialysis therapy, she received a cadaver kidney graft 11 months ago. All went very well and there is excellent function in the transplant kidney, which has a creatinine clearance of 70 ml/min. She has been given standard immunosuppressive therapy with azathioprine and prednisone. There was one acute rejection episode in the third week but this responded rapidly to a short course of steroids in very high dose.

Carol is now very well, but in the past two months her blood pressure has been rising and has now reached a level of 190/120. What is the cause of the hypertension?

In view of the fact that **Carol Owen's** original disease was pyelonephritis, there is hardly any question of recurrence of the original disease in the transplant kidney, as might be the case if the original disease had been a glomerulonephritis. You have also to consider the possibility of low grade, chronic rejection affecting principally the small arteries. This is unlikely with such excellent renal function and a normal urine, and it is ruled out when a biopsy of the grafted kidney proves normal. What would you advise now?

The most likely cause of **Carol Owen's** hypertension is stenosis of the arterial anastomosis, so you request angiography.

Figure 60 is an early film from the series and it shows a considerable stenosis at the anastomosis between the hypogastric artery and the donor renal artery. Would you now proceed to corrective surgery?

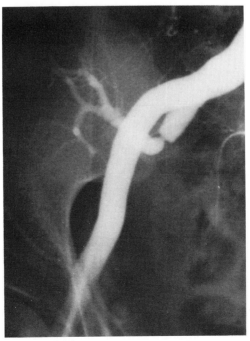

FIGURE 60. Carol Owen

It is, of course, vital to restore **Carol's** blood pressure to normal, but it may well be possible to do this with medical therapy and this should be tried first. Surgery may be necessary if the blood pressure proves difficult to control or if there is any serious increase in the stenosis.

Paul Tyler, age 24, a graduate student, was involved in an automobile accident last year. He had a nasty head injury, and was unconscious for four days. During that time he had an indwelling urethral catheter. Happily, he made a complete recovery and returned to his studies but he now complains of increasing difficulty in micturition, with a poor stream. He says also that he dribbles for some minutes after voiding. What do you think is the cause of his trouble?

Clearly there is obstruction of Paul Tyler's lower urinary tract. Much the most likely cause is urethral stricture, and this diagnosis is confirmed when instruments passed into the urethra meet an obstruction at the penoscrotal junction. Filiform bougies are negotiated through the narrow region, and the stricture is dilated. How do you view the future management of this case?

It would of course be possible to keep the stricture dilated by passing sounds at appropriate intervals, but naturally **Paul Tyler** does not like the idea of submitting to this procedure two or three times a year for the rest of his life, and he would much prefer some corrective surgery that would provide a permanent cure.

Before deciding on urethroplasty it is essential to know the full extent of the stricture, and so you request a retrograde urethrogram (Fig. 61). This reveals that the stricture at the penoscrotal junction is in fact very short and should be relatively simple to correct surgically. Notice the dilatation of the proximal urethra above the stricture.

The stricture was due to pressure necrosis caused by too large an indwelling catheter at the time of the head injury. Urethral problems after catheter drainage are all too common. To avoid such complications, you should not only use a catheter of nonreactive material such as silastic but also use the smallest catheter that will carry the traffic.

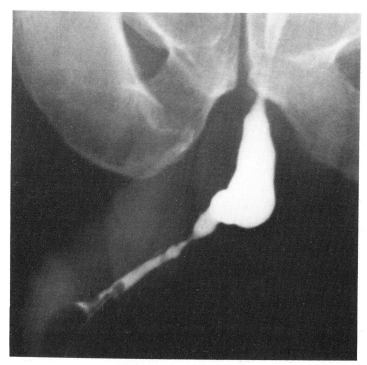

FIGURE 61.   Paul Tyler

Dinny Bray, a 26 year old singer with a rock group, complains of a dull pain in the right side of his abdomen. As so often happens in such cases, physical examination and routine lab studies are unrewarding. An upper GI series was normal so you decide, as the next step, to request an intravenous urogram.

This is the 10 minute film (Fig. 62) from **Dinny's** IVP. There are a few flecks of barium scattered through the colon. The obvious feature is a space-occupying lesion in the upper pole of the right kidney. The smooth, regular deformity of the upper calyces suggests solitary cyst rather than tumor. What do you propose next?

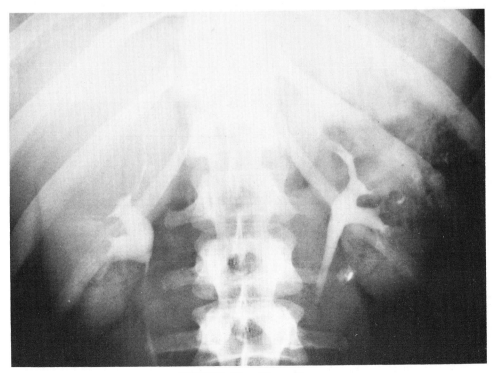

FIGURE 62. Dinny Bray

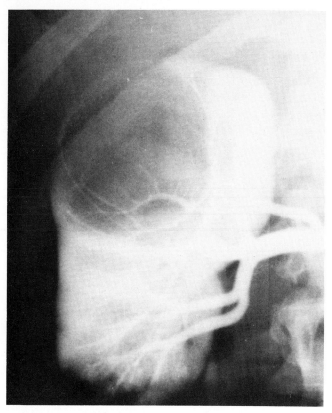

FIGURE 63. Dinny Bray

A good way to distinguish between cyst and tumor in the kidney is by selective renal angiography. This was done with **Dinny Bray**; Figure 63 is from the arteriogram phase and Figure 64 is the film of the nephrogram phase.

You can see that there are no tumor vessels, and the lesion is uniformly lucent and smoothly circular. It is a solitary cyst and quite harmless. Cyst puncture with injection of contrast medium would also be a useful technique.

Such cysts frequently produce no symptoms, but in the present case the cyst is likely to be responsible for *Dinny's* pain, and so it should be explored surgically and unroofed.

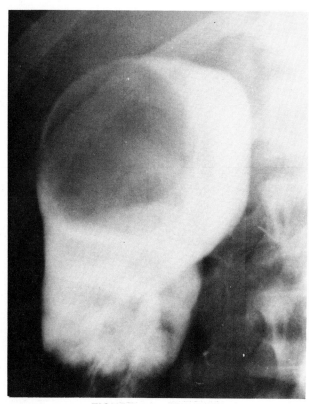

FIGURE 64. Dinny Bray

Baby Young has been a bare 30 hours in the world but clearly all is not well with him. He is a puny, mewling infant. Palpation of his abdomen reveals a cystic swelling rising out of the pelvis as high as the umbilicus. You suspect that the swelling is a distended bladder and when you press on it a few drops of urine trickle from the urethra. You also discover that he has passed very little urine since birth. What x-ray studies would you request?

In an adult your first thought would be to request an intravenous urogram, but in small children a *voiding cysto-urethrogram* is often more rewarding. A small catheter is passed easily into **Baby Young's** bladder and nearly 300 ml of urine is withdrawn. A water-soluble contrast medium is then injected through the catheter and spot films are taken.

The most striking feature of this film (Fig. 65) is that there is more contrast medium in the right kidney and upper right ureter than in the bladder. There is obviously gross reflux up the right ureter, and if you look closely you can see that the reflux continues from the middle and upper calyces into the collecting tubules. The parenchyma of the kidney is thinned down to little more than a half centimeter; this means that renal function is depressed.

Tubular function will be affected more than glomerular function, and concentrating ability is impaired, with the result that the kidney produces a large volume of dilute urine. In an infant this in turn introduces a grave risk of serious dehydration.

You can also see that the bladder is trabeculated, an indication of lower tract obstruction.

More contrast medium is introduced until it begins to leak alongside the catheter, which is then withdrawn, and more films are taken as the bladder tries to empty.

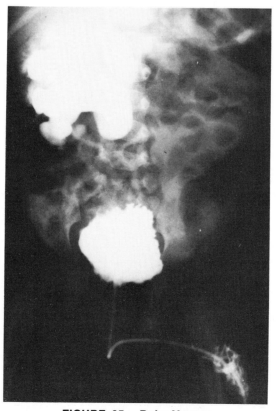

FIGURE 65. Baby Young

Figure 66 is **Baby Young's** voiding film. The bladder neck is so dilated, as is the first part of the urethra, that you cannot see where the bladder ends and urethra begins. The prostatic urethra is severely obstructed by congenital valves.

The resting films, A–P and lateral, taken after micturition (Figs. 67 and 68) show the gross distention of the right upper tract. Note how the ureter has become elongated and convoluted; this has an important bearing on treatment. Simple drainage of the bladder would not empty the atonic upper tract, and so the procedure of choice is cutaneous loop ureterostomy. At a later date the urethral valves will be removed by transurethral resection, and later still the ureterostomy will be closed.

What about the left kidney? It has not shown up in any of the films. You might perhaps suggest that the left ureterovesical junction has successfully resisted the back pressure but this is very unlikely. In fact, later IVP studies confirmed that *Baby Young's* left kidney was absent — congenital defects are often multiple.

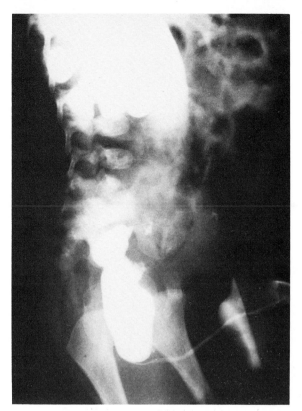

FIGURE 66. Baby Young

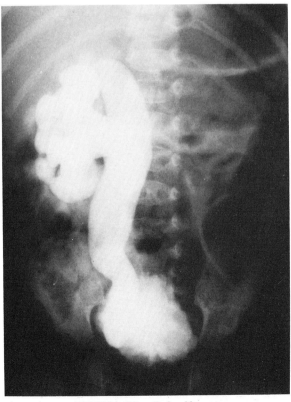

FIGURE 67. Baby Young

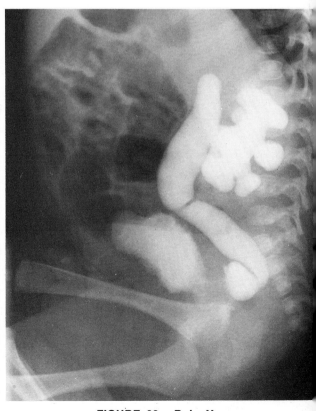

FIGURE 68. Baby Young

Mark Eager, a bustling advertising executive of 45 summers with a figure that speaks well for the size of his expense account, comes to the medical clinic for a checkup. He has never been ill and never consulted a physician, but recently he has been feeling unusually tired.

You find that *Mark's* blood pressure is 240/130, and examination of his optic fundi reveals papilledema and some nipping of the vessels. It is not easy to feel anything in his abdomen owing to the fat but you think that you can palpate both kidneys. Urinalysis shows 1+ albumin with a sediment containing some red cells, a few white cells and also granular casts. Hemogram and electrolytes are normal but the BUN is 35. How do you view the picture at this stage?

The presence of casts in **Mark Eager's** urine is positive evidence of renal parenchymal disease. Cells and albumin could derive from a lesion in the excretory pathway. The BUN indicates some degree of renal insufficiency. So far, you can consider the possibility that the renal disease is caused by the hypertension, or there may be a renal lesion causing the hypertension. However, you thought that you could feel both kidneys. If you can feel them in such a fat abdomen, they must be considerably enlarged. Does this suggest a definite diagnosis?

Full marks if you made a provisional diagnosis of polycystic disease of the kidneys. This is confirmed by **Mr. Eager's** IVP (Fig. 69). Both kidneys measure over 20 cm, and there is considerable distortion of the pelvicalyceal systems.

The all important principle in the management of *Mr. Eager's* disease is maintenance of the blood pressure at a normal level. Among other things, this will involve close supervision of salt balance, steering a careful course between the Scylla of salt excess and the Charybdis of salt depletion.

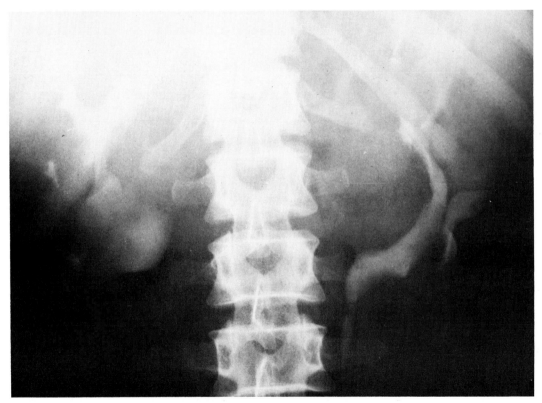

FIGURE 69. Mark Eager

Anna Ricci, 18 year old daughter of Italian immigrant Mr. Cacci Ricci, is brought by her father to the hospital with what seems to be a textbook attack of renal colic. She is extremely distressed, nauseated and sweating, with very severe pain radiating from her right flank to the right pubic region. Urinalysis confirms microscopic hematuria.

You relieve her pain with an analgesic and request a stat IVP. Figure 70 is the preliminary film. What do you make of it?

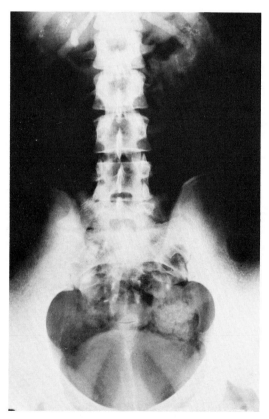

FIGURE 70. Anna Ricci

The most striking feature is the very large number of small opacities in the renal areas, with two much bigger opacities within the right kidney shadow. The film is not well centered: the upper part of **Anna's** left kidney is cut off, so you would like to see another plain film centered over the kidneys (Fig. 71). Now you have a clearer picture of the bilateral nephrocalcinosis. What are your thoughts at this stage?

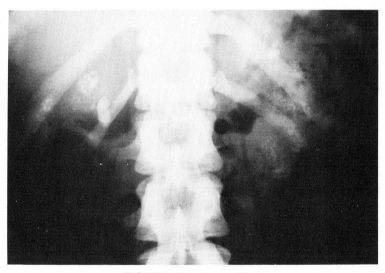

FIGURE 71. Anna Ricci

On **Anna Ricci's** new film, did you notice the pattern of the small snowdrifts of opacities? Especially on the left side, they are arranged in a way that corresponds to the medullary pyramids. Each little opacity is a tiny calculus in a cystic dilatation of a collecting tubule. The name that most accurately describes the condition is precalyceal canalicular ectasia but it is usually known as medullary sponge kidney. On the right side, the two bigger opacities are stones, one in an upper and one in a lower calyx, formed by ulceration of a tiny calculus from one of the small cysts.

In the 10 minute film of the IVP (Fig. 72) the major calyces, pelvis and upper ureter on the left side look normal. What about the right side? There does not appear to be any excretion of contrast medium. In this situation, it is a mistake to report "no function on the right side." It may be necessary to continue taking films for many hours (even 24 or 36) to get the true picture, as you can see if you turn to page 74.

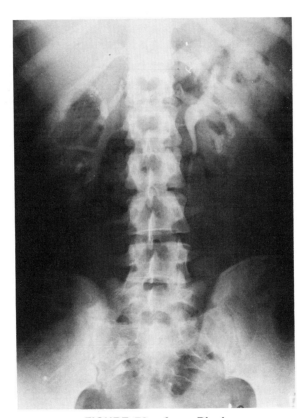

FIGURE 72. Anna Ricci

In **Anna Ricci's** 18 hour film (Fig. 73), you can see that there is no longer any contrast medium on the left side. On the right side there is a big stone obstructing the ureter at the level of the ischial spine. Why was this stone not visible in the preliminary film? Look at the detail from that film in Figure 74. There are in fact two opacities in the line of the right ureter but they are partly obscured because they lie over dense sacral bone. The lower of the two opacities is the ureteral stone, which has moved down to the ischial spine level by the time the 18 hour film was taken. The upper opacity is not a stone. If you look at it carefully in Figure

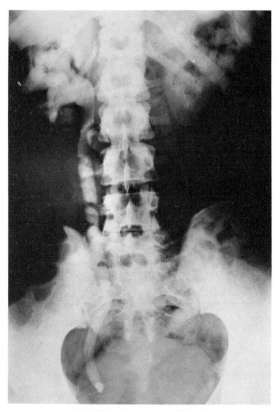

FIGURE 73. **Anna Ricci**

73, you can see that it lies outside the ureter.

The stone shifted a little further and then was removed from the intramural ureter by transurethral ureterolithotomy. It emerged that *Anna* had an older sister, Clara, who also had medullary sponge kidney but in Clara's case the renal condition was not complicated by calculi. Both sisters were losing excessive amounts of potassium in their urine (*Anna's* serum K was only 2.6 mEq per liter) and will have to take potassium supplements for life.

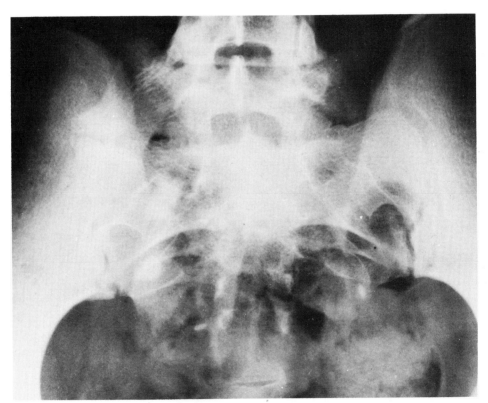

FIGURE 74. Anna Ricci

Ali Ramdan, age 30, is the Egyptian servant of a visiting Arab dignitary. He is brought to the Emergency Room in a state of great agitation complaining of hematuria which he first noticed two hours ago. His English is scanty so you cannot elicit much in the way of clinical history.

On physical examination you find no significant abnormality but urinalysis confirms that there is a large amount of blood in the urine.

Figure 75 is the preliminary film of **Ali Ramdan's** bladder area. What do you make of it?

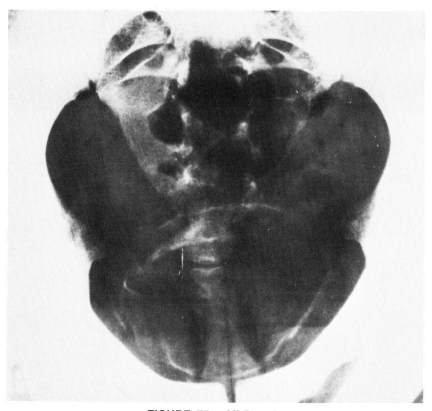

FIGURE 75. Ali Ramdan

Did you notice the thin line of calcification that seems to be outlining **Ali's** bladder? Figure 76 is a film of the bladder area from the pyelogram series, and this seems to confirm that the calcification was in fact in the wall of the bladder, and in addition you can see that there is a little dilatation of the lower end of each ureter.

What is your diagnosis?

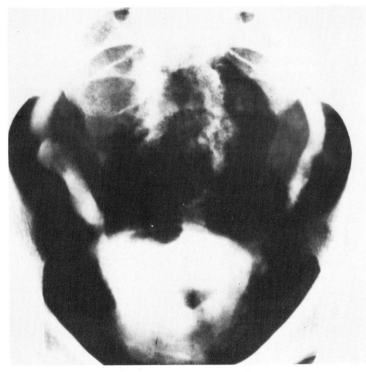

FIGURE 76. Ali Ramdan

Hematuria in any resident of a country where the disease is known to be endemic must arouse the suspicion of urinary schistosomiasis. The calcification in the wall of **Ali Ramdan's** bladder noted in the plain film is absolutely characteristic, and the diagnosis can be confirmed by finding the typical ova in the urine. You will have to do a cystoscopy to make sure there is no carcinoma in the bladder because malignant tumors of the bladder are a very common complication of urinary schistosomiasis.

For the treatment of this case, you will have to seek the help of experts in tropical medicine.

Thirty-two year old **Torry Pisa** has been investigated by his family doctor because of discomfort in the upper right quadrant of his abdomen. Physical examination and laboratory studies of blood and urine have shown nothing remarkable, but Figure 77 is the 10 minute film from his intravenous urogram. What do you make of it?

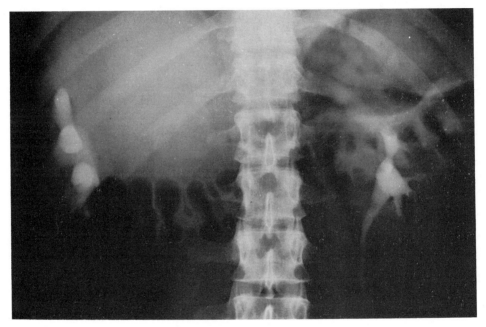

FIGURE 77.   Torry Pisa

The left kidney of **Torry Pisa** seems normal, but on the right side the kidney and urethra are leaning laterally, and it is reasonable to conclude that there must be some large mass causing this displacement.

You request selective renal angiography. Figure 78 is a film from the arteriogram phase and Figure 79 is the nephrogram phase from this series.

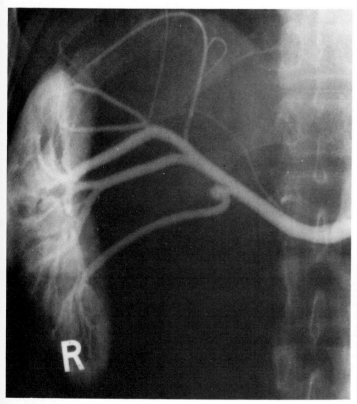

FIGURE 78. Torry Pisa

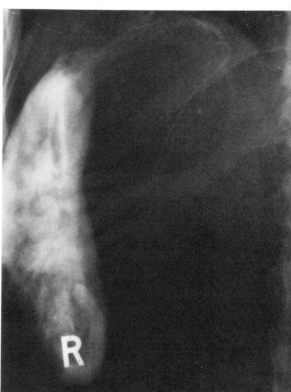

FIGURE 79. Torry Pisa

Torry Pisa's renal artery is enormously elongated and stretched out over a large mass closely applied to the medial border of the kidney, but there is no hint of vascularization of this mass and so it is likely to be a cyst rather than a tumor.

In fact, at this stage, exploratory surgery revealed that the mass was a gigantic hydronephrosis in the upper segment of a duplex kidney. It was quite a job to dissect this out without damaging the renal vessels stretched over it. The offending upper segment was, however, removed safely and *Mr. Pisa* made an uneventful recovery.

Jimmy King, a 29 year old gymnastics instructor, comes to your clinic complaining of painful swelling of the right testicle. He tells you that two weeks ago he slipped on the vaulting horse and hurt himself and that his right testicle has been painful and swollen ever since.

Physical examination reveals a fine specimen of athletic manhood. You confirm that the right testis is swollen to about twice its normal size and is distinctly tender. Routine laboratory studies and urinalysis are normal. Do you think that *Jimmy* has a traumatic hematocele?

With a history like **Jimmy King's** it is very dangerous to assume that the condition is simply the result of trauma. If *Jimmy* were a little younger you would give very strong consideration to the diagnosis of torsion of the testis, observing the important rule that any acute scrotum in a man under the age of 25 is a torsion of the testis until proved otherwise. Torsion can occur in older men, and must in fact be considered, but you would expect very much more pain with torsion. Tumor of the testis can also present as an acute scrotum and, as with torsion, a history of trauma may mislead you. Acute epididymitis can also present with such a history but it is usually possible to feel the massive swelling of the epididymis distinct from the testis, and in this case the swelling seems to be in the testis itself. Surgical exploration is urgently indicated.

In a case like that of **Jimmy King,** the scrotal contents are explored through an inguinal incision so that the spermatic cord can be clamped at the internal inguinal ring before the testis is handled; this is done to minimize the risk of tumor embolization. Frozen section of the testis revealed a seminoma, so the cord was divided at the internal ring and the testis was removed.

What is the further management of this patient?

In **Jimmy King's** case, detailed histologic examination of the tumor disclosed that it was a pure seminoma. This information lightens the gloom about the prognosis because seminoma is usually extremely radiosensitive. It is important now to establish the extent of any metastatic spread of the disease.

Testicular tumors tend to spread first along the path of the spermatic vessels to the para-aortic lymph nodes in the region of the renal vessels, and you may get valuable information from intravenous urography and from lymphangiography. Neither of these studies showed any abnormality in the present case, but Figure 80 is the chest x-ray. How do you interpret it?

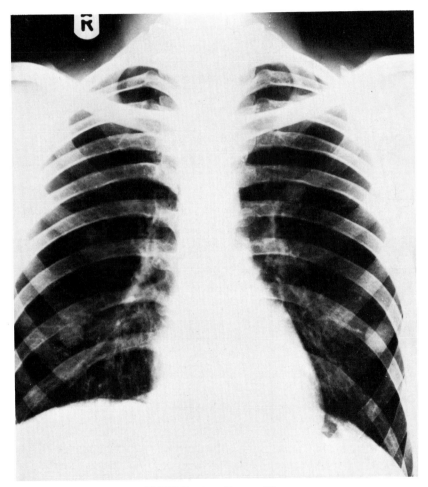

FIGURE 80.   Jimmy King

Round, clear cut densities are visible in both lung fields, and these are undoubtably metastases from the seminoma. It is worthwhile to attempt radiotherapy but the prognosis for **Mr. King** is obviously poor.

Cherry Rype, an 18 year old girl, is brought to the emergency room by friends who found her very sick in her apartment. She tells you that she has been unwell for more than a week, with pain in her right side, headache, and shivering. She thought that she had a bad chill and was dosing herself with aspirin. For the past two days she has been much worse and and has been vomiting.

Cherry is pale, with dark rings under her eyes, and looks very ill. Her temperature is 102.4°F. Examining her abdomen, you find a very large, acutely tender swelling occupying the whole of the upper right zone, and she is very tender in the right loin. The hemogram shows Hct 22, WBC 19,000. She is not able to provide a specimen of urine and catheterization reveals an empty bladder. Her BUN is 200. Supine and upright films of the abdomen (not illustrated) show a big soft-tissue mass in the right upper quadrant. What do you think is wrong? What will you do next?

The tender mass is probably a pyonephrosis but this is not enough to account for the uremia and the anuria unless it is a solitary kidney. In **Cherry's** case, there is little point in requesting an IVP, but retrograde pyelograms should give valuable information. Cystoscopy confirms that the bladder is empty. A catheter passes easily up the left ureter to the kidney; another catheter passed up the right ureter sticks at 18 cm. Contrast medium is injected up both ureteral catheters, and a spot film is taken. The film is reproduced on page 85. What is your opinion of this?

Cherry Rype's right ureter is deviated medially and is not seen above the fourth lumbar vertebra. Contrast material has entered only the upper part of the large right pyonephrosis. The rest of the pyonephrosis has been outlined by a broken line in Figure 81. If you waited some hours for the contrast material to diffuse you would probably get a pretty picture of the whole right kidney, but this would be an unjustifiable academic exercise. *Cherry's* life is at stake and treatment is urgent.

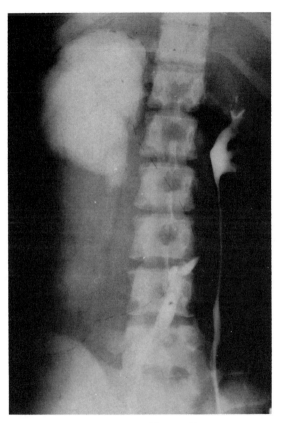

FIGURE 81. Cherry Rype

What about the left kidney? At a quick glance you might think it is normal, but look again. Did you notice how close it is to the vertebral column? It is, in fact, a very small kidney. The calyces are not crowded as in hypoplasia; it is probably contracted as a result of glomerulonephritis.

So we seem to have double pathology —an old glomerulonephritis and secondary sepsis in a congenital hydronephrosis on the right side. How will you treat *Cherry* now?

Two things must be done immediately for **Cherry Rype.** The right pyonephrosis must be drained; this is a simple matter of inserting a big tube, and it can be done with local analgesia. Secondly, with this degree of uremia in a hypercatabolic patient, dialysis is essential — among other reasons, to correct the severe metabolic acidosis that must be present.

Cherry's subsequent progress was, perhaps, surprising. When the tube was inserted, over two liters of thick pus were evacuated from the pyonephrosis. After three days, the draining fluid changed to clear urine. The left kidney did not make any significant contribution but the caricature of a kidney on the right side recovered sufficiently to keep *Cherry* in reasonable health for another two years before renal replacement therapy became necessary.

Lucy Small, age 9, is brought by her parents for a second opinion on the management of her hypertension. Two years ago *Lucy* woke one morning with a moderately severe headache. An alert family doctor took *Lucy's* blood pressure and found it abnormally high. After some investigation, hypotensive drugs were prescribed. Recently, Mr. and Mrs. Small have been getting worried because *Lucy* needs bigger and bigger doses of her drugs and yet the blood pressure is not well controlled. They have been told that *Lucy's* hypertension is due to chronic pyelonephritis affecting both kidneys.

Lucy is a pleasant, intelligent girl. She is 52 inches tall and weighs 63 pounds—normal figures for her age. You are alarmed to find the BP 220/160. Ophthalmoscopy reveals grade II hypertensive retinopathy, and the apex beat lies in the sixth left intercostal space, one inch lateral to the midclavicular line. There is a systolic murmur all over the precordium. Left ventricular hypertrophy is confirmed by chest x-ray and EKG.

Urinalysis shows the presence of RBCs and granular casts. Urine protein output is 1.6 gm in 24 hours. The BUN is 28 and serum creatinine 2.2. Hemoglobin is 9.4.

You naturally request an IVP for Lucy Small. Figure 82 is the 15 minute film from the IVP series. The contrast is poor because of the diminished renal function. Both kidneys are rather small, especially the left (note how close the left kidney is to the vertebral column; this is always a sign of a very small kidney). Look again at the left kidney. The contrast is greater in the lower calyces than in the upper,

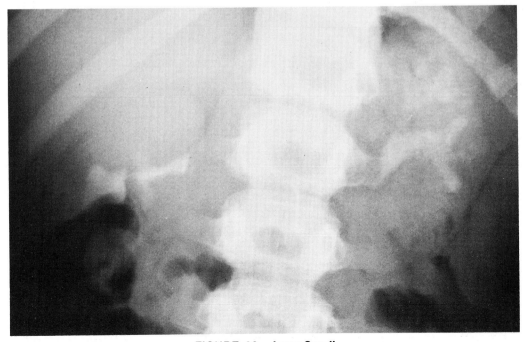

FIGURE 82. Lucy Small

and there is a very short distance between the calyces and the surface of the kidney. On the right side some calyces seem to be missing. The uppermost visible calyx is pointing almost directly medially and has the classic swallowtail appearance of segmental hypoplasia of the kidney.

Segmental hypoplasia is a developmental anomaly that may affect part or all of one kidney or parts of both kidneys; it is very frequently associated with severe hypertension.

In this case, the condition is much better displayed by renal angiography, and you can see some of these pictures below and on page 89.

Figure 83 is from the nephrogram phase of **Lucy Small's** renal arteriograms. Look at the right kidney first and notice that the upper third of this kidney shows much more densely than the remainder of the kidney, although there are mottled patches of density in the lower part of the kidney. Look very closely at the lower pole of the right kidney and you can see a tiny nubbin of renal tissue. The left kidney shows the same sort of changes, but the entire kidney is much smaller.

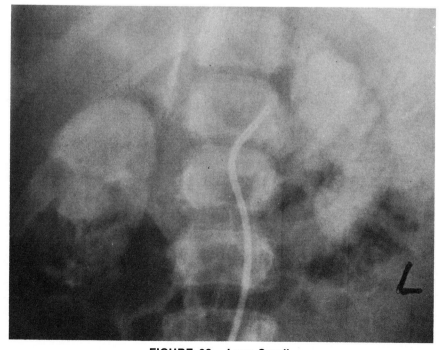

FIGURE 83. Lucy Small

Figure 84 shows a view of the right kidney in the arteriogram phase and here you can see very clearly the tiny nubbin of tissue at the lower pole and the irregularity of the outline of the kidney.

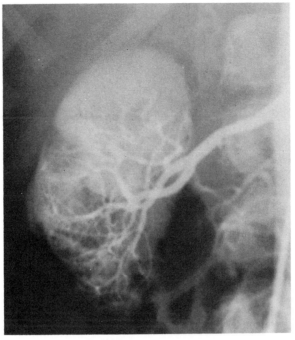

FIGURE 84. Lucy Small

Figure 85 is a slightly later film of the left kidney; it shows very well the deep notches corresponding to the hypoplastic segments.

How do you suggest that *Lucy's* problem should be managed?

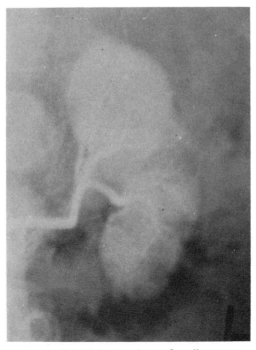

FIGURE 85. Lucy Small

Lucy Small's hypertension is very severe and not at all controlled by medical treatment. This is a sinister situation, all the more so because it will produce progressive nephroangiosclerosis in the relatively normal parts of the kidneys, and this must lead to renal failure and death. If, as may happen, the condition were confined to one kidney you could solve the problem very simply by removing that kidney. In some cases of bilateral disease, the hypoplasia affects only parts of each kidney and it is possible to remove the hypoplastic segments with restoration of blood pressure to normal.

In the present case, the disease is very widespread in both kidneys, and so the problem cannot be solved by any direct attack on the kidneys themselves.

The situation is desperate. If nothing can be done, *Lucy* is doomed. One possibility remains and that is to interrupt the renin-angiotensin pathways by removing both adrenal glands.

Following bilateral adrenalectomy, *Lucy's* blood pressure returned to normal. She is, of course, maintained on a small daily dose of steroid. One year after surgery, the blood pressure was still normal and the heart size had returned to normal. The retinal signs had also disappeared and renal function was slightly improved.

Bernie Villa, age 10, is referred by his doctor for investigation of attacks of left loin pain recurring over a period of two months. *Bernie* is otherwise healthy with no other symptoms and has no history of previous illness. You note a pink, papular rash on his face and upper chest. His mother tells you that this rash has been present for some years. There is no other clinical abnormality, and routine lab studies on blood and urine are also normal. Because of the recurrent attacks of loin pain you request an IVP.

Figure 86 is the 30 minute film from **Bernie's** IVP series. On the left side, function is very poor but you can make out a large renal pelvis, and no contrast medium has entered the left ureter. You might be inclined to think that *Bernie's* left loin pain was due to congenital hydronephrosis, but did you look carefully at the right kidney? On the right side, the calyces and pelvis seem to be rotated downward by a space-occupying lesion in the upper half of the right kidney.

In fact this drooping-flower appearance is very like that seen in cases of ectopic ureter, where the ectopic ureter comes from an upper segment which functions too poorly to show up on IVP. However, in such cases, the poorly functioning upper segment is usually small, whereas you can get a definite impression that there is a considerable amount of tissue in the right kidney above the visible calyces. How would you proceed now?

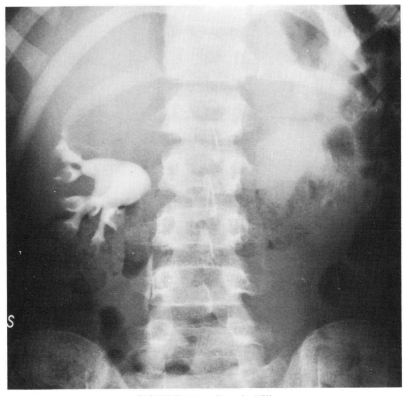

FIGURE 86. Bernie Villa

A micturating cystogram of **Bernie Villa** was normal, with no evidence of reflux. You might elucidate the situation on the left side by retrograde uretero-pyelograms but this will not help you to solve the problem of the right side, so you request renal angiography.

Figure 87 is one of the pictures from the arteriogram phase on the right side. There is a large lucent area occupying the entire upper part of the right kidney. Do you think that this is a simple cyst?

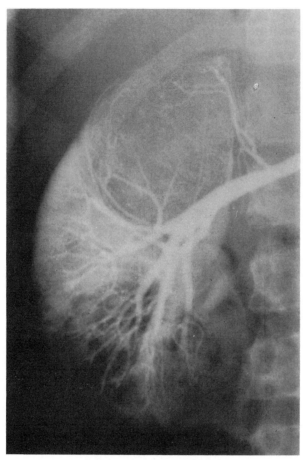

FIGURE 87.   Bernie Villa

There are too many small vessels going into this lesion to regard it as a simple cyst. On **Bernie's** original film one can also see areas of slight pooling of the contrast medium. This is the picture of a relatively avascular tumor rather than a cyst. Now look at the rest of the right kidney in the same figure. Can you see several tiny cysts in the rest of the kidney, and also a certain amount of mottling suggesting irregular pooling of contrast medium? These features are more obvious when you look at the nephrogram phase (Fig. 88).

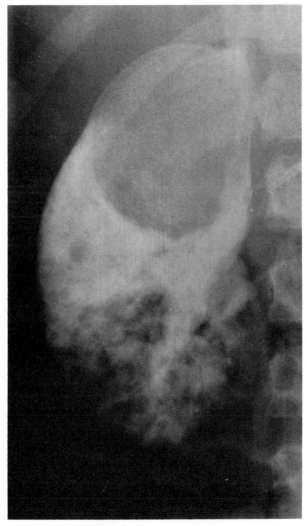

FIGURE 88.   Bernie Villa

Figure 89 is from the early arteriogram phase of the left side and you can see that the vessels to the lower pole give the appearance of being stretched over some ill-defined space-occupying lesion.

You might at this stage be inclined to think in terms of bilateral renal tumors, but look again at the rash on *Bernie's* face.

This is a case of tuberous sclerosis. The brain is often affected in this disease and so you will request an EEG and brain scan. These, in fact, proved normal.

Biopsy of the skin lesions on the chest showed altered dermal collagen and several immature hair structures, findings compatable with a diagnosis of tuberous sclerosis. The right kidney was explored, and a biopsy of the tumor mass occupying the entire upper pole confirmed the diagnosis of tuberous sclerosis. The hydronephrosis on the left side was due to compression by a similar mass in the lower part of the left kidney.

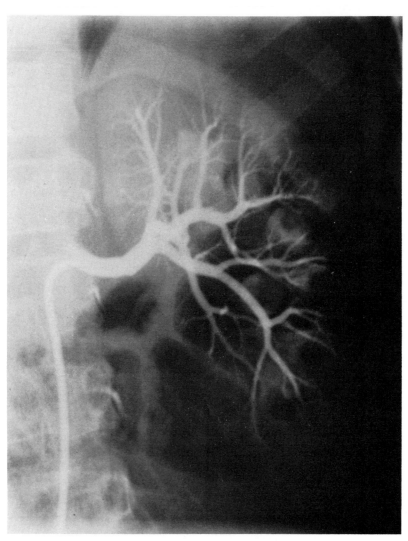

FIGURE 89. Bernie Villa

Elsa Flood, an 18 year old hospital secretary, has been having recurrent attacks of urinary infection with chills and pain in the left loin. Figure 90 is a picture from her IVP series. How do you interpret it?

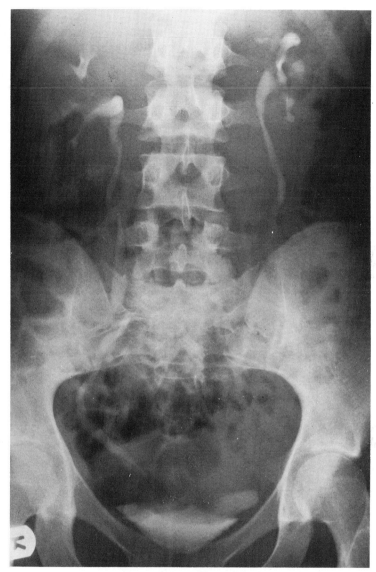

FIGURE 90. Elsa Flood

Elsa Flood

The left kidney is small. The right kidney is grossly normal but seems a little large, as if it has undergone compensatory hypertrophy. Returning to the left side, you might think that this was a relatively unremarkable pyelonephritic kidney, but if you look more closely you will see that the uppermost calyx seems to be missing.

At cystoscopy you find a normal bladder with normal ureteral orifices. To get a clearer picture, you pass a catheter up the left ureter and take a retrograde pyelogram (Fig. 91). This shows (what can, in fact, be seen in the IVP) a curious streak of contrast medium passing medially from the uppermost visible calyx.

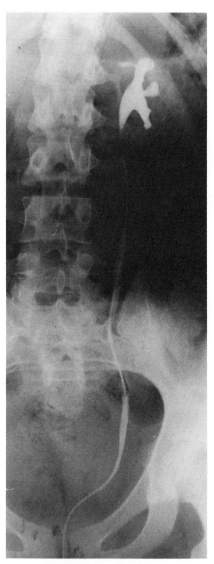

FIGURE 91. Elsa Flood

Elsa Flood

Even though the ureteral orifices looked absolutely normal at cystoscopy you request a micturating cystogram and are rewarded by an unexpected dividend. Figure 92 is an oblique film taken when the bladder was nearly empty. There is a huge ectopic ureter opening into the upper part of the urethra and this has been filled with contrast medium by reflux during micturition. There is no urinary incontinence because the ureter opens into the urethra above the external sphincter.

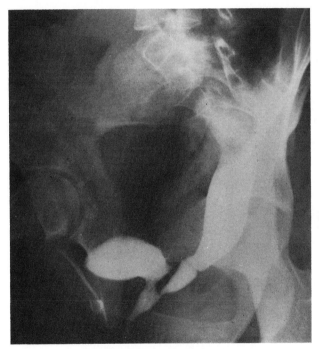

FIGURE 92. Elsa Flood

You now repeat the endoscopy, doing what you should have done the first time — taking a careful look at the urethra as you pass the instrument in. This step is all too often overlooked. The procedure should be cystourethroscopy rather than cystoscopy. In fact, you can easily see the large opening of the ectopic ureter in the left side of the upper urethra. You pass a catheter into this opening and another catheter up the normal left ureter and inject contrast medium into both, producing the picture that you see in Figure 93.

To cure *Elsa's* recurrent infection, it would be necessary to remove not only the upper segment of kidney but also the entire ectopic ureter. The ureter will have to be taken right down to its junction with the urethra. If any stump is left it will continue to act as a urethral diverticulum and a source of continued infection.

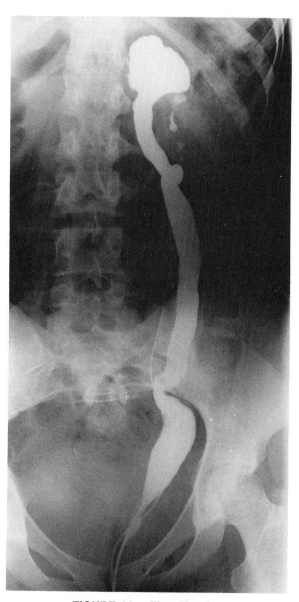

FIGURE 93. Elsa Flood

Zoe Zhivago, the 74 year old mother of a well known doctor, had a total cystectomy for bladder carcinoma five years ago. She is now living in your area and comes to you because she has been told that she should have a checkup every year.

You are a little surprised to find that her urine was diverted into the intact colon (ureterosigmoidostomy) but *Mrs. Zhivago* tells you that she has been very well ever since her surgery. She has no complaints. She passes urine from the rectum approximately every three or four hours and has normal control.

The particular problem with this form of urinary diversion is the risk of hyperchloremic acidosis caused by absorption of chloride ions from the large intestine. You request full blood chemistry studies and find that the creatinine and BUN levels are normal. The plasma chloride is a little high and the plasma bicarbonate is slightly below normal. There is also a risk of potassium loss in these patients so you are happy to find a normal plasma potassium.

Clinical examination and a chest x-ray give no evidence of metastatic disease. Do you need any further studies or can you now reassure *Mrs. Zhivago* that all is well?

In every type of urinary diversion it is as well to do a limited IVP at least once a year. If you look at Figure 94, which is the 10 minute film from **Mrs. Zhivago's** IVP series, you will see why. The right kidney seems normal, although the right ureter is a little dilated in its full length. On the left side there is no visible contrast medium. The most likely explanation for this is a silent obstruction. There are several other things to note in this picture: the osteoarthritis of the spine; the irregular vertical line immediately to the left of the lumbar vertebrae, indicating calcification in the abdominal aorta; and the oval opacity high on the left side, showing between the eleventh and twelfth ribs. How do you interpret this opacity?

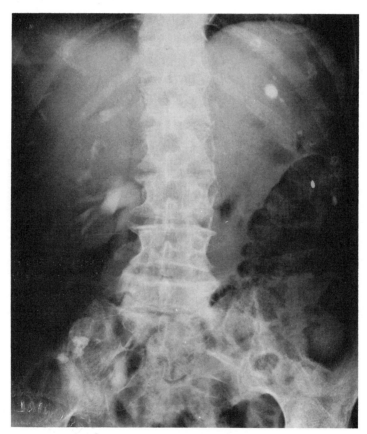

FIGURE 94. Zoe Zhivago

The clear definition and perfect oval shape should give you the clue. This is a tablet lying in **Mrs. Zhivago's** stomach. It would be a good idea to ask her what medication she is taking. It may be a sodium bicarbonate tablet prescribed by a previous doctor to combat the mild acidosis.

Look again at the right kidney. In the uppermost calyx you can see a filling defect. Now look at Figure 95, which is an oblique view of the right kidney and ureter, and you can see a large oval filling defect in the right ureter just to the right of the fourth lumbar vertebra, with a small circular filling defect above it. These filling defects represent bubbles of gas that have refluxed up the right ureter from the intestine.

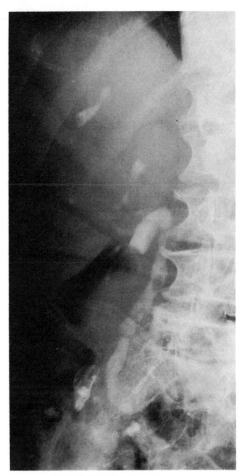

FIGURE 95.   Zoe Zhivago

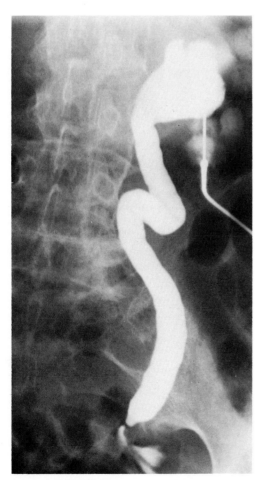

FIGURE 96.   Zoe Zhivago

The only way to get more information about the radiologically silent left kidney is to do an antegrade pyelogram, in other words to insert a needle into the left renal pelvis and inject contrast medium. This was done and you can see one of the subsequent pictures in Figure 96. This shows very clearly a gross dilatation of the left ureter, with a stricture where the ureter joins the intestine. Occlusion is not complete, as is shown by the fact that some of the contrast medium has passed on into the intestine.

This case illustrates some of the problems of urinary diversion, especially diversion into the intestine. On the right side the ureterocolic anastomosis is, so to speak, too wide open and there is reflux from the intestine into the ureter. On the left side a stricture has been produced and the left kidney has been destroyed without any symptoms.

There is not much point now in doing anything about the left side, although it may be necessary to remove the left kidney if *Mrs. Zhivago* should develop pyonephrosis on that side. Should the right side be left alone or should it be converted to a cutaneous ureterostomy? This is a difficult question to answer. Probably the best solution is to keep the situation under careful review. A single-film IVP taken 30 minutes after injection of contrast medium every four to six months should alert you in time if trouble is developing on the right side. You do not want to submit *Mrs. Zhivago* to unnecessary surgery and give her a cutaneous stoma if she could carry on as she is. Equally you must not let the right kidney get into the same sort of trouble that has developed on the left side.

INDEX